ATKINS DIET BOOK FOR BEGINNERS 2024

Unlock the power of nourishing and empowering low-carb recipes for weight loss and healthy living.

DR EMILY THOMPSON

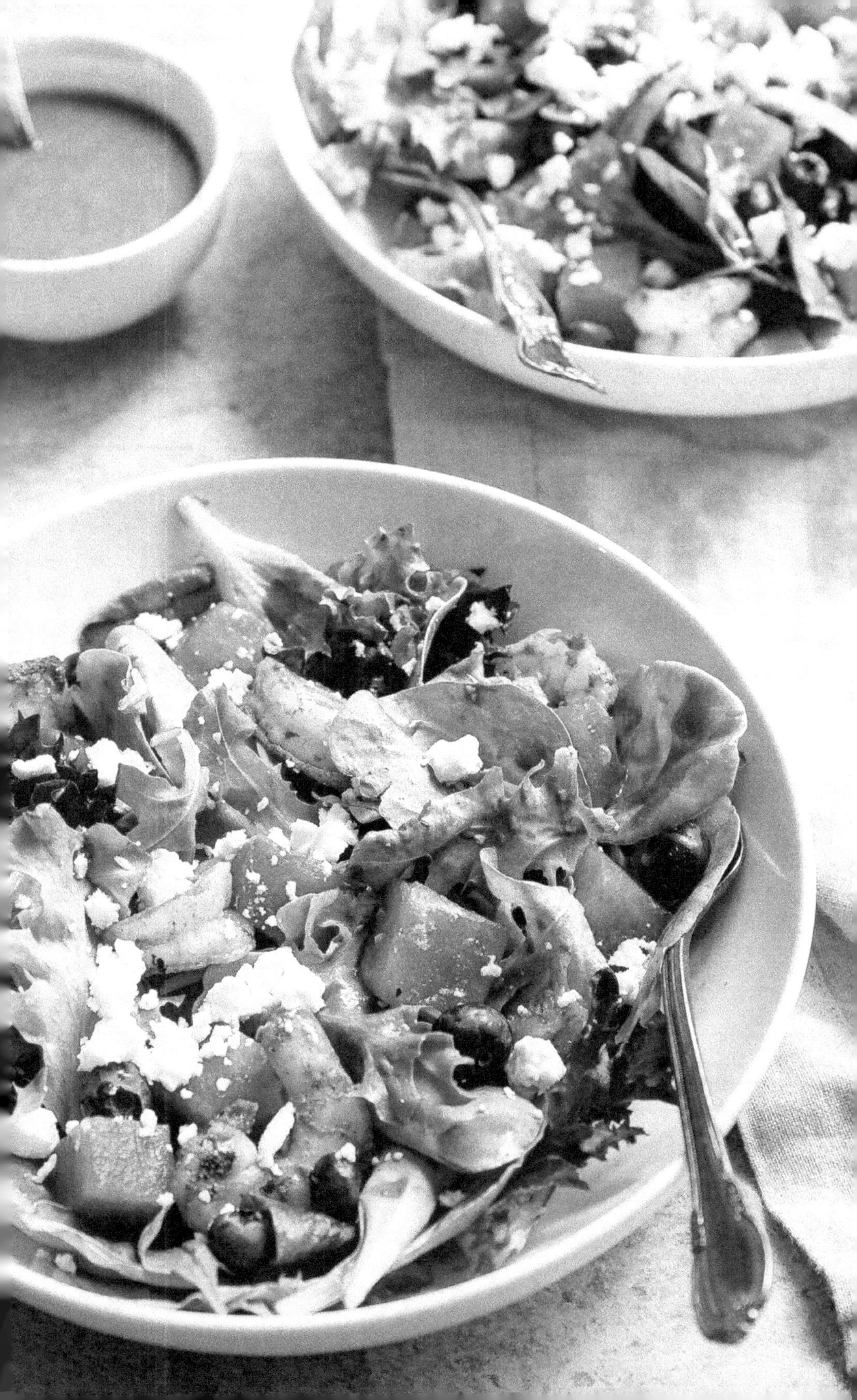

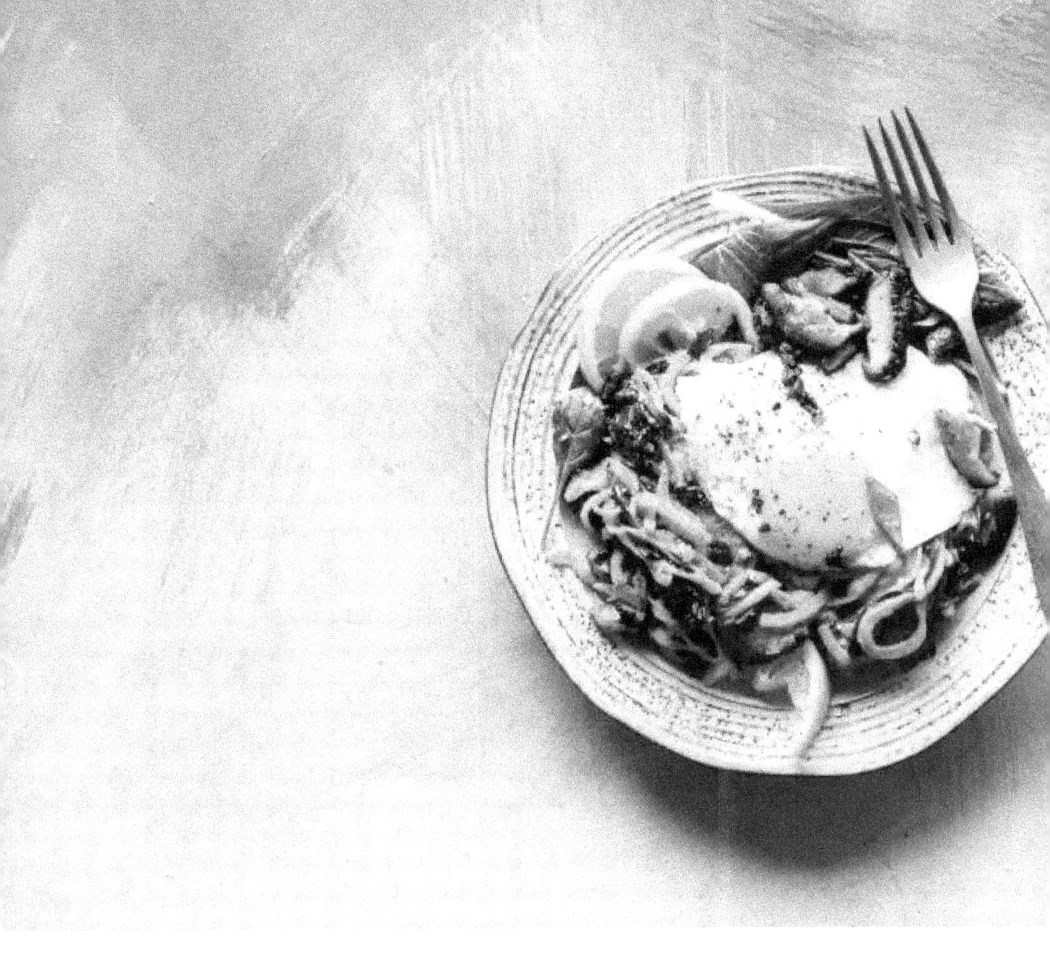

TABLE OF CONTENT

Introduction

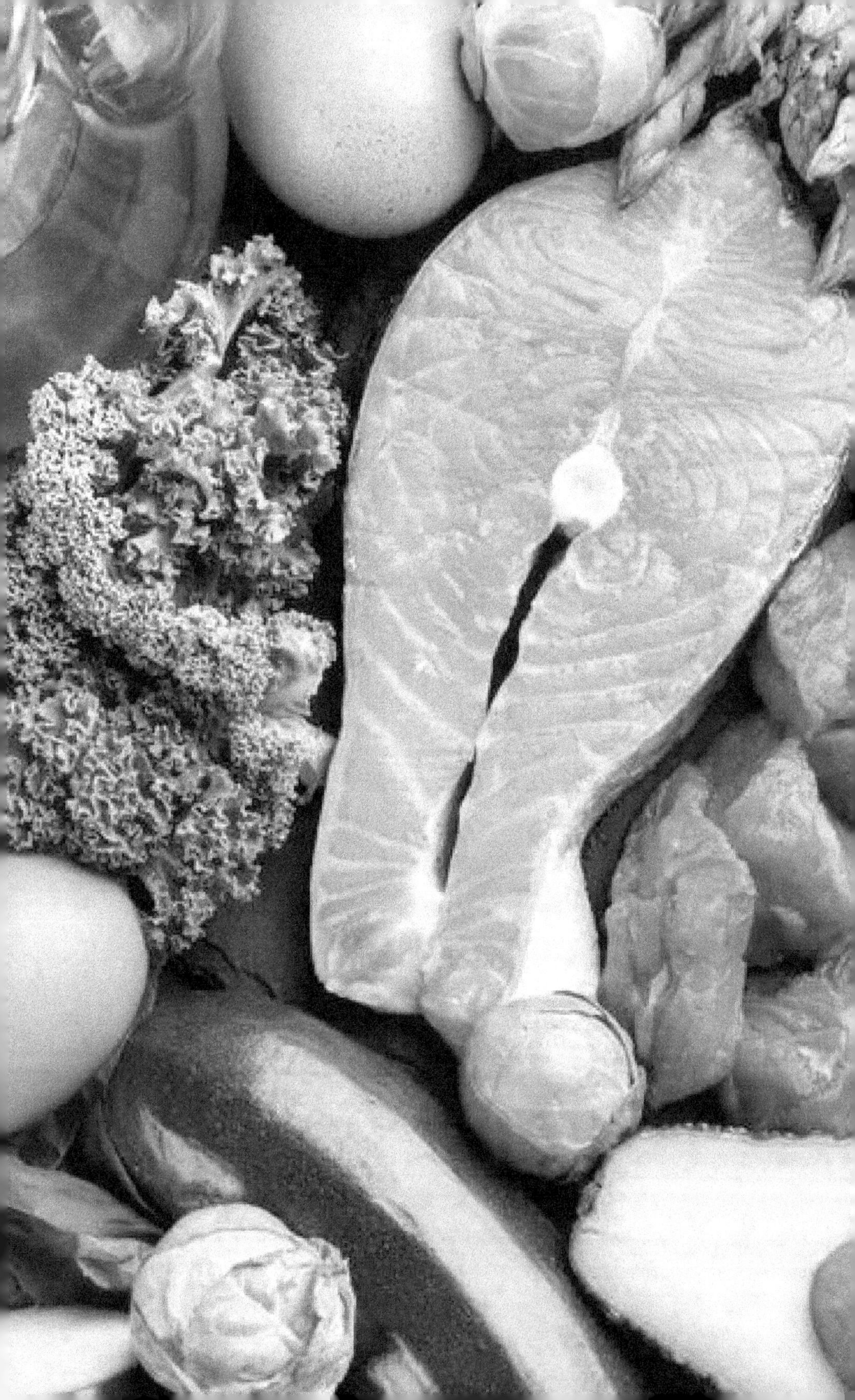

INTRODUCTION

In the quiet moments between dusk and dawn, when the world seems to hold its breath, there exists a unique space—the space of transformation. It's a space where dreams take root and whispers of change weave through the air. It was in such a space, decades ago, that Dr. Robert Atkins stood on the precipice of a dietary revolution that would touch the lives of millions.

Let me transport you to that moment, to the year 1972. Dr. Atkins, a visionary cardiologist, faced a world entrenched in the belief that low-fat diets were the path to health. But Dr. Atkins dared to dream differently. He saw a world where the shackles of conventional wisdom could be broken, where the journey to wellness wasn't paved with deprivation but with a profound understanding of the body's intricate dance with food.

In the early days, his ideas faced skepticism. Critics dismissed him as a maverick, but undeterred, he forged ahead, driven by a belief that would alter the course of nutrition forever. He unveiled the Atkins Diet—a paradigm shift that would echo through the years, transcending the barriers of doubt and skepticism.

Fast forward to today, to the year 2024. The Atkins Diet has evolved, not just as a weight-loss solution but as a beacon of empowerment and well-being. It's a journey that transcends the boundaries of dieting and steps into the realm of a lifestyle—a lifestyle that beckons you to unlock the power within yourself.

Now, imagine yourself standing at the threshold of your own transformation. Maybe you're yearning for a change, for a healthier version of yourself. Perhaps you've tried diets that promised the moon but left you grasping at unfulfilled dreams. The year 2024 is your moment, and the "Atkins Diet Book for Beginners 2024" is your guide.

This isn't just a book; it's an invitation to a journey of self-discovery and nourishment. It's a journey where every page is a step toward understanding the beauty of the food you eat, the strength within your choices, and the transformative power of the Atkins lifestyle.

As you turn the pages, you'll not only uncover the science behind the Atkins Diet but also stories—stories of triumph, resilience, and the quiet victories of everyday warriors who, like you, stood at the crossroads of change.

This book is more than a manual; it's a companion. A companion that holds your hand through the aisles of the grocery store, whispers encouragement in moments of doubt, and celebrates each milestone, no matter how small.

So, dear reader, whether you're standing at the beginning of your journey or seeking a fresh start, know that within these pages lies a tapestry of possibility. The "Atkins Diet Book for Beginners 2024" is an offering, an embrace, and an echo of the dreams that stirred in the heart of Dr. Robert Atkins all those years ago.

Are you ready to step into the space of transformation? The journey awaits, and the first chapter begins now. Welcome to a year of possibility, empowerment, and the unlocking of your own extraordinary potential. Welcome to "Atkins Diet Book for Beginners 2024."

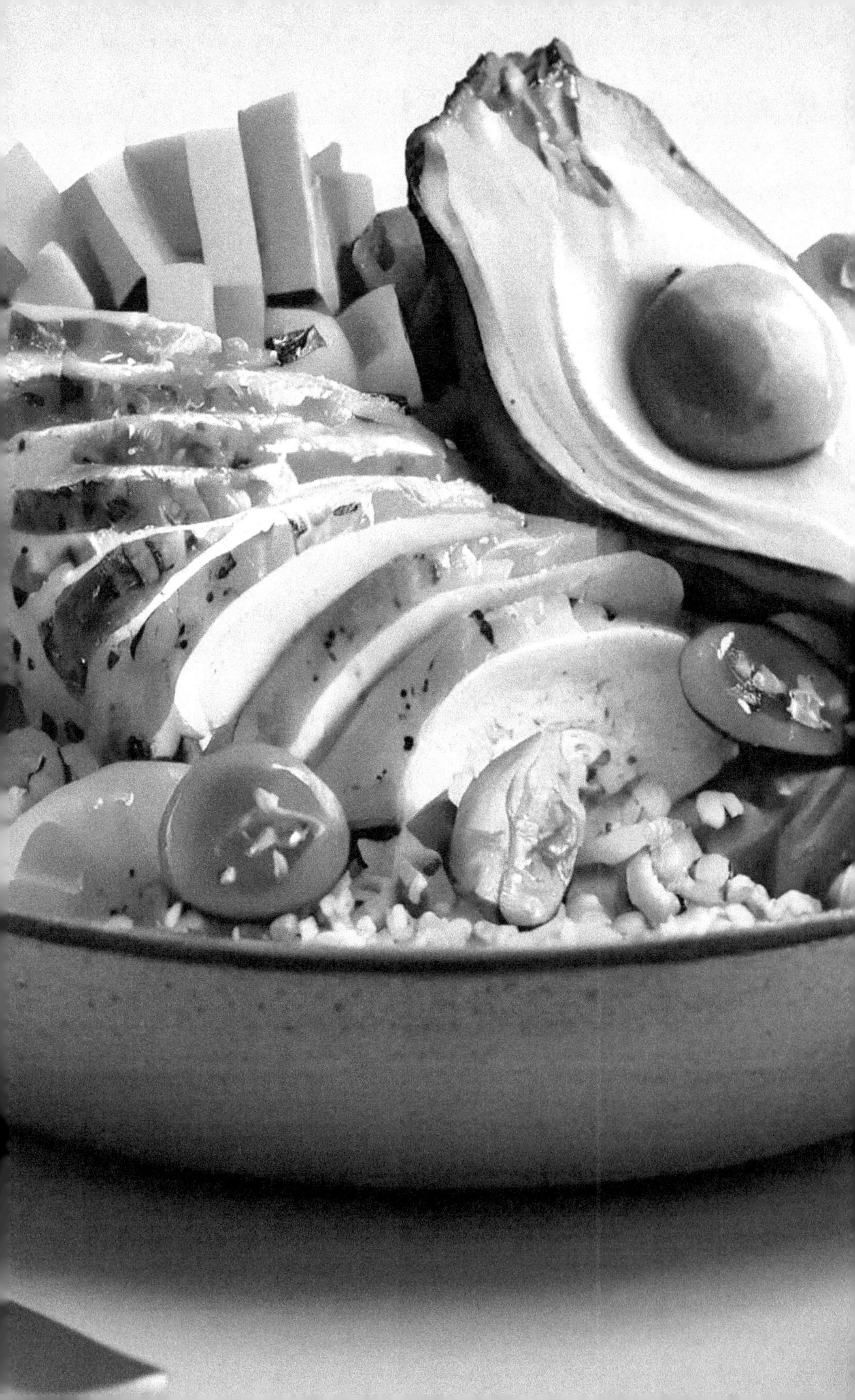

Brief History and Evolution of The Atkins Diet

The Atkins Diet, born out of the pioneering work of Dr. Robert Atkins in the early 1970s, has undergone a fascinating evolution, transforming from a controversial dietary approach to a widely recognized and respected method for weight loss and overall health improvement. Dr. Atkins, a cardiologist, challenged the conventional wisdom of his time, advocating a low-carbohydrate lifestyle to combat obesity and promote well-being.

In the initial years, the Atkins Diet faced skepticism from the medical community, as the prevailing narrative emphasized low-fat diets for weight management. Dr. Atkins, however, believed that restricting carbohydrates, particularly refined sugars, could trigger a metabolic state called ketosis, where the body utilizes stored fat for energy. The induction of ketosis became a cornerstone of the Atkins Diet, setting it apart from conventional dietary practices.

As the years progressed, several clinical studies began validating the efficacy of the Atkins Diet in weight loss and improving metabolic markers. The diet's emphasis on protein and healthy fats, coupled with reduced carbohydrate intake, proved to be a successful formula for many individuals. The evolving scientific landscape increasingly supported Dr. Atkins' initial theories, leading to a shift in public perception.

The Atkins Diet's popularity surged in the late 1990s and early 2000s as a growing number of success stories emerged. Celebrities and everyday individuals alike credited the diet for their remarkable weight loss achievements and improved overall health. This widespread acceptance prompted a reconsideration of dietary guidelines and contributed to a broader conversation about the role of carbohydrates in our daily nutrition.

In recent years, the Atkins Diet has continued to adapt to the evolving understanding of nutrition and dietary science. The emphasis has expanded beyond weight loss to encompass overall health and well-being. The diet's flexibility and personalized approach have made it relevant to a diverse audience, and its principles continue to be integrated into various contemporary low-carb lifestyles.

Overview of the Book's Purpose and What Readers can Expect.

Welcome to "Atkins Diet Book for Beginners 2024," a comprehensive guide designed to unlock the power of nourishing and empowering low-carb recipes for weight loss and healthy living. This book is more than just a compilation of recipes; it's your companion on the journey to understanding, embracing, and successfully implementing the Atkins Diet in the year 2024.

Our primary aim is to demystify the Atkins Diet, making it accessible to beginners and offering a fresh perspective for those familiar with its principles. We understand that embarking on a new dietary journey can be both exciting and challenging, and our book is crafted to be your reliable source of information and inspiration.

Understanding the Atkins Diet: The book begins with a thorough exploration of the Atkins Diet's principles and phases. We break down the science behind the diet, explaining the significance of each phase and how carb restriction induces the metabolic state of ketosis. This section serves as your foundation, ensuring you comprehend the "why" behind the dietary choices you'll be making.

Getting Started: To set you up for success, we provide practical guidance on preparing for your Atkins journey. From setting realistic goals to stocking your kitchen with essential items, this chapter equips you with the tools you need to navigate the initial stages effectively. We believe that a well-prepared start enhances your chances of long-term success.

Meal Planning and Recipes: Arguably the heart of the book, the chapter on nourishing low-carb recipes introduces you to a delectable array of dishes tailored for beginners. We emphasize variety, taste, and simplicity, recognizing that enjoying your meals is crucial for sustained adherence to the diet. Weekly meal plans further simplify your dietary choices, making it easier to integrate the Atkins lifestyle into your routine.

Nutritional Guidance: Understanding the role of protein and fats is essential for a balanced Atkins Diet. In this section, we delve into the specifics, providing practical tips for achieving nutritional balance. We want you to feel confident in your food choices, knowing that you're nourishing your body optimally.

Navigating Challenges: No dietary journey is without its challenges. Cravings, plateaus, and social situations can be stumbling blocks. Our book addresses these common hurdles head-on, offering strategies and insights to keep you on track. By acknowledging and preparing for challenges, you'll be better equipped to overcome them.

Health Benefits Beyond Weight Loss: While weight loss is a significant goal, the Atkins Diet offers a multitude of health benefits. In this chapter, we explore how the diet positively impacts cardiovascular health, blood sugar control, and more. Real-life success stories and testimonials add a personal touch, inspiring you to envision the broader spectrum of well-being the Atkins lifestyle can offer.

Fitness and Exercise: Complementing your dietary choices with physical activity is crucial for holistic health. We guide you through integrating exercise into your routine, ensuring a well-rounded approach to your wellness journey.

Sustainability and Long-Term Success: The Atkins Diet is not a short-term fix but a lifestyle. In this chapter, we provide tips for transitioning between phases and maintaining your results. Our goal is to empower you to make the Atkins Diet a sustainable and enjoyable part of your life.

Resources and Tools: To enhance your experience, we've compiled a toolkit featuring supplementary materials, shopping lists, and online resources. Quick-reference charts make it easy to navigate key aspects of the Atkins Diet, ensuring you have the support you need at your fingertips.

Conclusion: As you reach the end of this book, we recap the key takeaways and offer words of encouragement for the journey ahead. Your success is our success, and we want you to feel motivated and confident as you embrace the Atkins lifestyle.

Appendix: Glossary of terms and quick-reference charts in the appendix provide valuable resources for ongoing reference, making the book a comprehensive guide that you can return to whenever needed.

Engagement and Community Building: We invite you to share your progress and experiences on social media using our dedicated hashtag. Additionally, consider joining our private Facebook group where you can connect with fellow readers, share tips, and find support throughout your Atkins journey.

Promotion and Post-launch Engagement: To help you on your journey, take advantage of limited-time promotions, and bonuses for early buyers. We're committed to ongoing engagement, responding to your reviews and feedback. Periodic updates and additional content releases will keep the book relevant and valuable long after your initial read.

Welcome to "Atkins Diet Book for Beginners 2024." Your journey begins here, and we're excited to be your trusted companion every step of the way.

Detailed Explanation of the Atkins Diet Phases

The Atkins Diet is characterized by its distinctive approach to weight loss and overall health, achieved through a series of carefully designed phases. Each phase serves a specific purpose, gradually introducing and adjusting the intake of carbohydrates to achieve optimal results. Let's delve into a detailed explanation of the Atkins Diet phases:

1. Induction Phase:

- **Objective:** The primary goal of the Induction Phase is to transition the body into a state of ketosis. Ketosis occurs when the body shifts from using carbohydrates as its primary source of energy to burning stored fat. This phase kickstarts the weight loss process.

- **Duration:** Typically lasts for two weeks, but individuals may choose to extend it based on their goals and how their body responds.

- **Carbohydrate Intake:** Extremely limited to 20-25 grams of net carbs per day, primarily derived from non-starchy vegetables. High-fiber, nutrient-dense carbs are encouraged.

- **Foods to Emphasize:**
  - Protein-rich foods such as meat, poultry, fish, and eggs.
  - Healthy fats, including olive oil, avocado, and nuts.
  - Leafy green vegetables.

- **Foods to Avoid:**
    - High-carb foods like grains, sugar, and starchy vegetables.
    - Fruits (except small amounts of berries).

2. Balancing Phase (Ongoing Weight Loss):

- **Objective:** Transition from rapid weight loss to a more gradual and sustainable pace. This phase helps determine an individual's Critical Carbohydrate Level for Losing (CCLL), the maximum amount of daily carbs that allows continued weight loss.
- **Duration:** Until you are within 10 pounds of your target weight.
- **Carbohydrate Intake:** Gradual increase by 5-10 grams per week. This phase involves finding the right balance of carbs for continued weight loss.
- **Foods to Emphasize:**
    - Diverse low-carb vegetables.
    - Additional nuts, seeds, and berries.
    - Controlled portions of other low-carb foods.
- **Foods to Avoid:**
    - Foods that may impede weight loss progress.

3. Pre-Maintenance Phase:

- **Objective:** Prepare for the Maintenance Phase by slowing down weight loss and finding the Critical Carbohydrate Level for Maintenance (CCLM). This phase helps identify the carb threshold at which weight remains stable.
- **Duration:** When you are within 5-10 pounds of your target weight.

- **Carbohydrate Intake:** Incremental increases to continue finding the right balance for weight maintenance.

- **Foods to Emphasize:**

  - A wider variety of fruits, legumes, and whole grains.

  - Continued focus on nutrient-dense, low-carb foods.

- **Foods to Avoid:**

  - Foods that may lead to weight gain.

4. Maintenance Phase:

- **Objective:** Sustain the achieved weight loss and overall health improvements. This phase allows for a flexible but controlled intake of carbohydrates to maintain the desired weight.

- **Duration:** Ongoing, making the Atkins lifestyle a permanent way of eating.

- **Carbohydrate Intake:** Adjusted based on individual tolerance, allowing for a sustainable and enjoyable diet.

- **Foods to Emphasize:**

  - A balanced mix of low-carb and higher-carb foods.

  - Focus on overall health and well-being.

- **Foods to Avoid:**

  - Excessive intake of refined carbohydrates.

- **Hydration:** Throughout all phases, staying well-hydrated is crucial for overall health and can aid in mitigating some side effects of the diet.

- **Supplementation:** Depending on individual needs, supplementation of vitamins and minerals may be recommended, especially in the initial phases.

- **Individual Variability:** It's important to note that the duration and specifics of each phase may vary based on individual responses, health goals, and lifestyle factors.

The Atkins Diet's phased approach provides a structured framework for individuals to achieve their weight loss goals while gradually incorporating a variety of foods to maintain a sustainable and healthy lifestyle. As with any diet, consulting with a healthcare professional or a registered dietitian is recommended before starting the Atkins Diet, especially for those with pre-existing health conditions.

Importance of Carb Restriction and the Science behind Ketosis.

1. **Insulin Regulation:**

   - Carbohydrates, especially refined sugars and starches, cause a spike in blood glucose levels. The body responds by releasing insulin to help transport glucose into cells for energy or storage. Continuous high-carb intake can lead to insulin resistance, a condition associated with obesity and type 2 diabetes. Carb restriction helps regulate insulin levels, promoting better blood sugar control.

2. **Enhanced Fat Utilization:**

   - When carbohydrate intake is restricted, the body shifts to an alternative energy source—fat. This process encourages the breakdown of stored fat into ketones, which can be used by the body and brain for fuel. Carb restriction thus facilitates efficient fat utilization, aiding in weight loss and metabolic health.

3. **Appetite Regulation:**

   - High-carb diets, particularly those rich in refined sugars, often lead to rapid spikes and crashes in blood sugar levels, contributing to increased hunger. Carb restriction, especially in the context of low-glycemic and nutrient-dense foods, helps stabilize blood sugar levels, reducing cravings and promoting a sense of fullness, ultimately supporting weight management efforts.

4. **Metabolic Flexibility:**

   - Restricting carbs encourages the body to become metabolically flexible, capable of efficiently using both carbohydrates and fats for energy. This flexibility is beneficial for overall health and performance, especially during periods of fasting or low-carb intake.

5. **Inflammation Reduction:**

   - Some studies suggest that high-carb diets, particularly those with an imbalance of omega-6 to omega-3 fatty acids, may contribute to systemic inflammation. Carb restriction, combined with a focus on anti-inflammatory foods, has been associated with reduced inflammation markers, potentially benefiting conditions linked to chronic inflammation.

6. **Improvement in Metabolic Syndrome Markers:**

   - Carb restriction has been shown to improve various markers associated with metabolic syndrome, including reduced triglyceride levels, increased HDL cholesterol, and improved blood pressure. These improvements contribute to a decreased risk of cardiovascular diseases.

The Science behind Ketosis:

1. **Shift in Fuel Source:**

   - In a typical Western diet, the primary source of energy is carbohydrates. When carb intake is restricted, glycogen stores in the liver and muscles are depleted. The body then shifts to using stored fat for energy, a process known as lipolysis. The byproducts of fat breakdown are ketones, which become the primary fuel source during ketosis.

2. **Ketone Production:**

   - Ketones, specifically beta-hydroxybutyrate (BHB), acetoacetate, and acetone, are produced in the liver as fats are broken down. These ketones can cross the blood-brain barrier and serve as an efficient energy source for the brain, especially during periods of low glucose availability.

3. **Enhanced Fat Oxidation:**

   - Ketosis enhances the oxidation of fatty acids for energy production. This metabolic state promotes the breakdown of stored fat, leading to weight loss. The increased utilization of fat for energy is a key factor in the success of low-carb and ketogenic diets for those aiming to shed excess body fat.

4. **Appetite Suppression:**

   - Ketones, particularly BHB, have been associated with reduced appetite. The mechanisms behind this appetite-suppressing effect are not fully understood but may involve interactions with neural pathways that regulate hunger.

5. **Stabilization of Blood Sugar Levels:**

- Ketosis results in a more stable and lower level of blood glucose, reducing the need for insulin secretion. This can be particularly beneficial for individuals with insulin resistance or type 2 diabetes, helping to improve blood sugar control.

6. **Anti-Inflammatory Effects:**

   - Some studies suggest that ketosis may have anti-inflammatory effects, potentially mediated through the suppression of pro-inflammatory pathways. This anti-inflammatory property may contribute to the observed improvements in various health markers during ketosis.

7. **Maintenance of Lean Body Mass:**

   - Contrary to concerns about muscle loss during ketosis, research indicates that the body can spare lean muscle mass. Adequate protein intake, which is a crucial component of the Atkins Diet, helps preserve muscle tissue even during periods of carbohydrate restriction.

In summary, carb restriction and the induction of ketosis play integral roles in reshaping the body's metabolic landscape. By tapping into the body's ability to utilize fat for fuel and producing ketones, individuals following low-carb approaches like the Atkins Diet may experience a range of health benefits, including weight loss, improved metabolic markers, and enhanced overall well-being. As with any dietary approach, individual responses may vary, and consulting with a healthcare professional is advisable, especially for those with pre-existing health conditions.

CHAPTER THREE
PREPARING FOR SUCCESS

Setting Realistic Goals and Expectations

Embarking on the Atkins Diet is more than a journey to shed a few pounds; it's a commitment to a lifestyle change that can transform your relationship with food and your overall well-being. As you step into this chapter, take a moment to reflect on your goals—what brought you here and what you aspire to achieve. The foundation of success lies in setting realistic goals and managing expectations.

Understanding Your Why: Before diving into the practical aspects of the Atkins Diet, it's crucial to identify your motivations. Are you looking to lose weight, manage blood sugar, or enhance your overall health? Each person's journey is unique and defining your "why" provides the compass for your path ahead. It could be regaining confidence, improving energy levels, or addressing specific health concerns. Whatever your reason, let it be the North Star guiding your efforts.

SMART Goals: Once you've clarified your overarching objectives, it's time to translate them into SMART goals—Specific, Measurable, Achievable, Relevant, and Time-bound. For instance, instead of a vague goal like "lose weight," a SMART goal would be "lose 10 pounds in the next eight weeks by following the Atkins Diet and incorporating regular exercise." This specificity not only sharpens your focus but also allows for tangible milestones along the way.

Understanding the Phases: As you set your goals, familiarize yourself with the different phases of the Atkins Diet. The induction phase, balancing phase, pre-maintenance, and maintenance phases each serve a unique purpose.

Acknowledge that the journey involves progression through these phases, each requiring adjustments in your approach. Setting short-term goals aligned with each phase ensures a structured and achievable path.

Managing Expectations: The Atkins Diet is not a one-size-fits-all solution. While many individuals experience significant weight loss and health improvements, it's essential to recognize that results vary. Factors such as metabolism, activity levels, and individual responses to dietary changes influence outcomes. Instead of fixating solely on the scale, celebrate non-scale victories—increased energy, improved mood, or enhanced mental clarity.

Creating Milestones: Break down your long-term goals into smaller, manageable milestones. These milestones act as checkpoints, allowing you to celebrate progress along the way. For example, if your goal is to lose 30 pounds, set milestones for every 5 pounds lost. Recognizing and celebrating these achievements reinforces your commitment and motivates you to push forward.

Adjusting Goals as Needed: Flexibility is key. As you progress through the Atkins Diet, reassess your goals periodically. You might find that your initial objectives evolve based on your experiences and results. Embrace the adaptability of your journey, adjusting goals to align with your changing needs and aspirations.

Visualizing Success: Visualization is a powerful tool in goal setting. Envision the healthier, happier version of yourself. Picture the activities you'll enjoy, the confidence you'll exude, and the positive impact on your overall well-being. This mental imagery serves as a constant reminder of your objectives, reinforcing your commitment to success.

In setting realistic goals and managing expectations, remember that the Atkins Diet is not a sprint but a marathon—a sustainable lifestyle change that unfolds over time. Embrace the journey, and success will follow.

23

Tips for Grocery Shopping and Kitchen Essentials

With your goals set and expectations managed, the next crucial step in preparing for success on the Atkins Diet is conquering the realm of grocery shopping and ensuring your kitchen is well-equipped for the journey ahead. These tips will guide you through the aisles and help you stock your kitchen with essentials that align with the principles of the Atkins lifestyle.

Creating a Low-Carb Grocery List: The foundation of your Atkins journey lies in the foods you bring into your home. Begin by crafting a comprehensive grocery list that prioritizes low-carb, nutrient-dense options. Include a variety of vegetables, lean proteins, healthy fats, and dairy products. Familiarize yourself with the carb counts of different foods, opting for those that align with the phase you're in.

Navigating the Perimeter: In most grocery stores, the perimeter is home to fresh produce, meat, seafood, and dairy—a haven for Atkins-friendly foods. Focus your attention on these sections to ensure you're choosing whole, unprocessed options. Fresh, colorful vegetables, lean cuts of meat, and quality dairy products are staples that should dominate your shopping cart.

Reading Labels Mindfully: As you explore the interior aisles, where packaged and processed foods reside, hone your label-reading skills. Check for hidden sugars, additives, and high-carb content. Choose products with minimal ingredients and, whenever possible, opt for whole, unprocessed alternatives. The more natural the food, the better it aligns with the principles of the Atkins Diet.

Stocking Up on Low-Carb Pantry Staples: Certain pantry staples form the backbone of a low-carb kitchen. These include:

- **Oils and Vinegars:** Olive oil, coconut oil, and balsamic vinegar.

- **Spices and Herbs:** Enhance flavor without added carbs.

- **Nuts and Seeds:** Great for snacking and adding crunch to meals.

- **Flours and Alternatives:** Almond flour, coconut flour, and other low-carb alternatives.

- **Condiments:** Mustard, mayonnaise, and sugar-free dressings.

Prioritizing Fresh Produce: Vegetables are a cornerstone of the Atkins Diet. Opt for a colorful array of non-starchy vegetables such as leafy greens, broccoli, cauliflower, and bell peppers. These provide essential vitamins, minerals, and fiber while keeping carb intake in check.

Protein Power: Ensure your protein sources are varied and high-quality. Incorporate lean meats, poultry, fish, eggs, and tofu into your meals. Protein is crucial for satiety and muscle maintenance, supporting your overall health and weight loss goals.

Smart Dairy Choices: Dairy can be part of a balanced Atkins diet but choose wisely. Select full-fat or low-fat options, avoiding those with added sugars. Greek yogurt, cheese, and butter can be included in moderation.

Meal Planning for Success: Plan your meals ahead of time, considering the specific phase of the Atkins Diet you're in. This not only streamlines your grocery shopping but also ensures that your kitchen is stocked with the necessary ingredients for your chosen recipes. Meal planning minimizes the chances of impulsive, carb-heavy choices.

Investing in Kitchen Tools: Equip your kitchen with tools that simplify the preparation of low-carb meals. Consider items such as a spiralizer for vegetable noodles, a quality blender for smoothies, and a food scale for accurate portion control. These tools enhance the variety and creativity of your meals, making the Atkins lifestyle enjoyable and sustainable.

Staying Hydrated: Don't forget the importance of hydration in your Atkins journey. Water should be your primary beverage, but herbal teas, black coffee, and sugar-free flavored water can add variety. Adequate hydration supports overall health and can help mitigate some common side effects during the initial phases.

In essence, successful navigation of grocery shopping and kitchen essentials for the Atkins Diet involves a thoughtful, informed approach. By prioritizing whole, low-carb foods, mastering label reading, and keeping your kitchen stocked with essential tools, you lay the groundwork for a successful and sustainable journey towards your health and wellness goals. The choices you make in the grocery store and the items you keep in your kitchen are pivotal components of your commitment to the Atkins lifestyle.

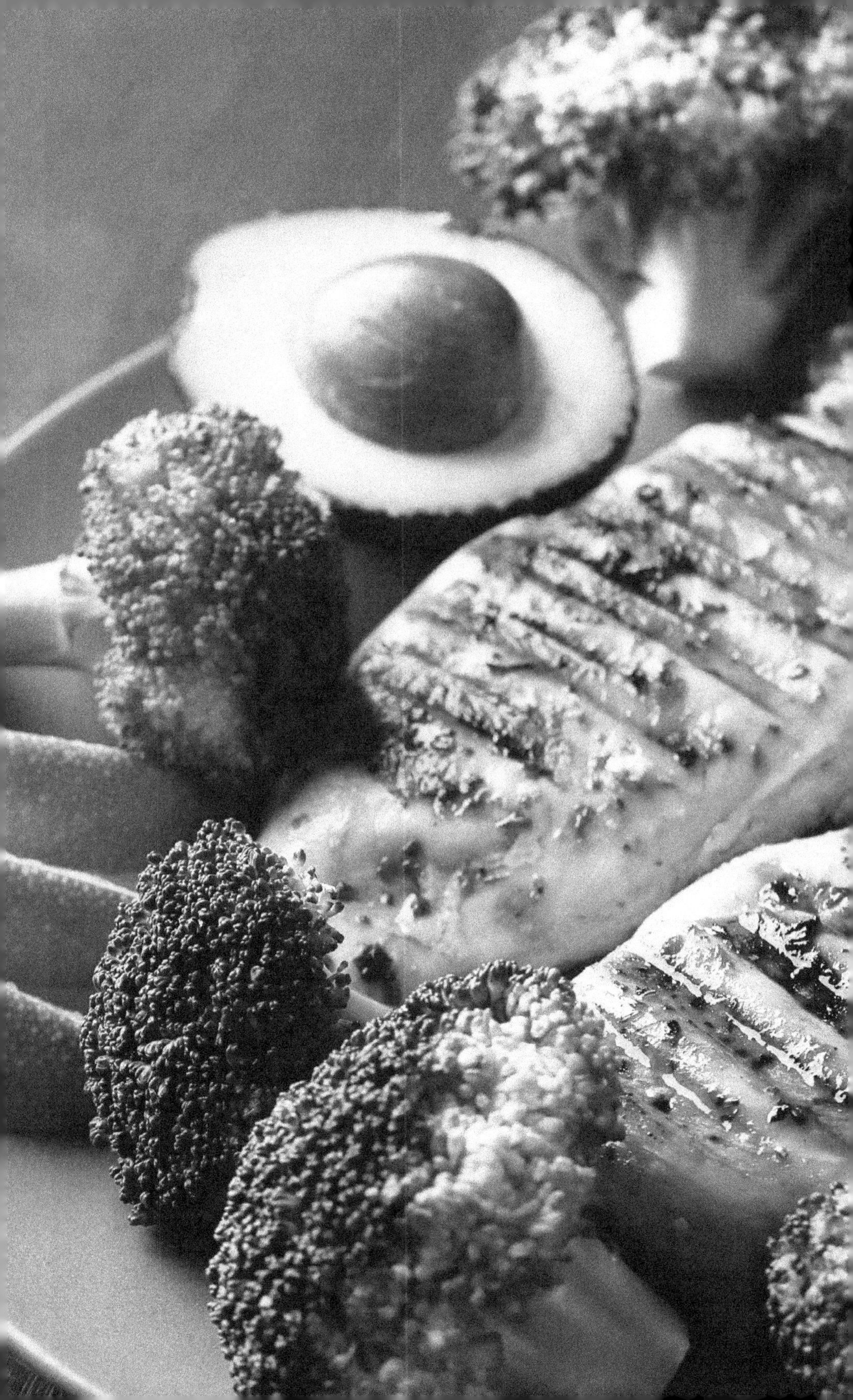

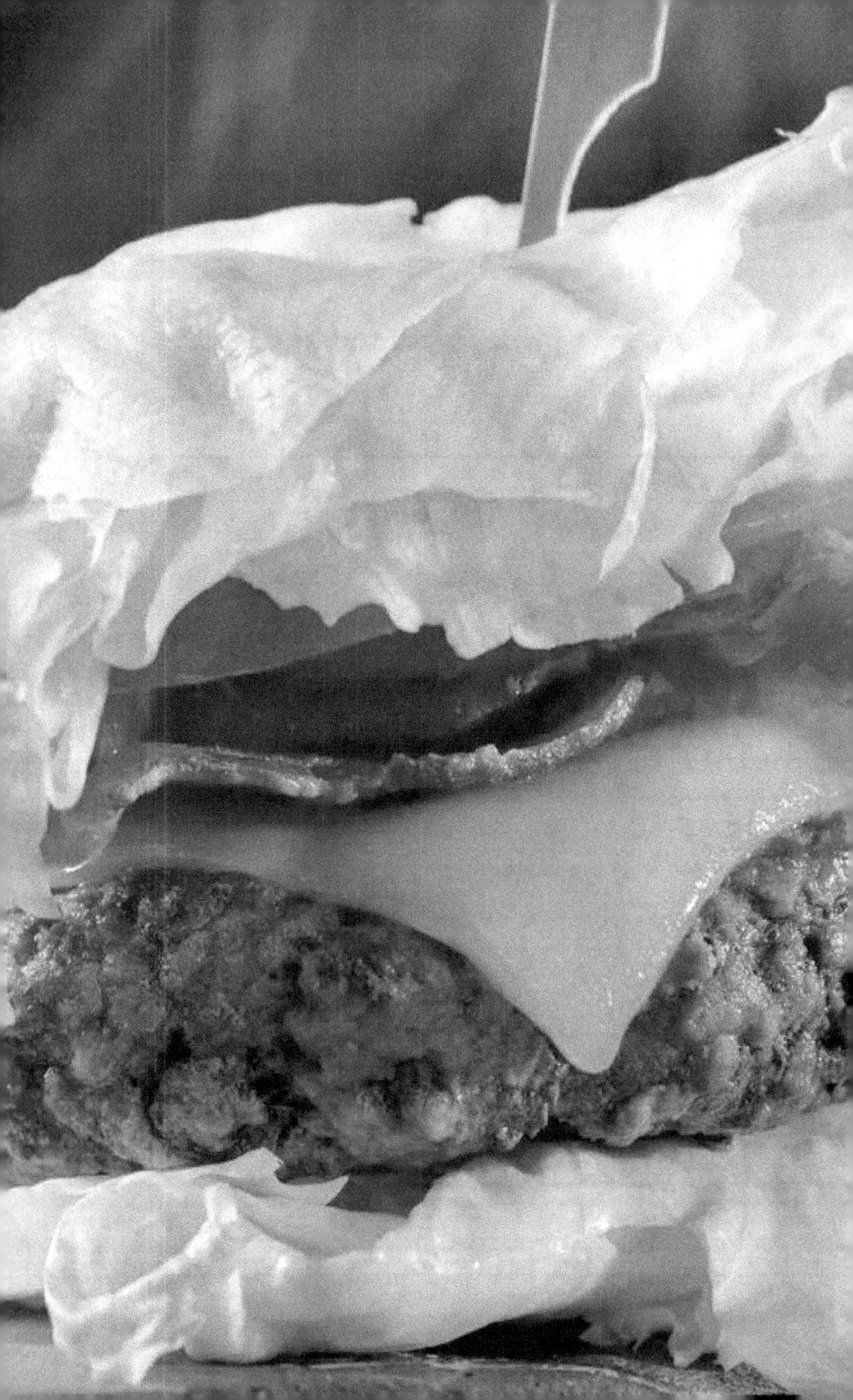

Beginner-Friendly Recipes for All Phases of the Atkins Diet

Embarking on the Atkins Diet is an exciting culinary journey that opens the door to a world of delicious, low-carb possibilities. Whether you're in the Induction Phase, the Balancing Phase, Pre-Maintenance, or Maintenance, these beginner-friendly recipes are crafted to suit all phases while embracing the principles of the Atkins lifestyle.

1. Spinach and Feta Omelette (All Phases)

Ingredients:

- 3 large eggs
- 1 cup fresh spinach, chopped
- 2 tbsp feta cheese, crumbled
- Salt and pepper to taste
- 1 tbsp olive oil for cooking

Instructions:

1. In a bowl, whisk the eggs until well combined.
2. Heat olive oil in a non-stick pan over medium heat.
3. Add chopped spinach to the pan and sauté until wilted.
4. Pour the whisked eggs over the spinach, letting them set slightly.
5. Sprinkle feta cheese evenly over the eggs.

6. Once the edges set, carefully fold the omelette in half.

7. Cook until the eggs are fully set, and the cheese is melted.

8. Season with salt and pepper to taste.

9. Serve hot and enjoy a protein-packed, low-carb breakfast.

Nutritional Information (per serving):

- Calories: 320

- Protein: 20g

- Fat: 25g

- Carbohydrates: 4g

- Fiber: 2g

- Net Carbs: 2g

2. Grilled Chicken Salad with Avocado (All Phases)

Ingredients:

- 6 oz grilled chicken breast, sliced

- 2 cups mixed salad greens

- 1/2 avocado, diced

- Cherry tomatoes, halved

- Cucumber, sliced

- Red onion, thinly sliced

- 2 tbsp olive oil

- 1 tbsp balsamic vinegar

- Salt and pepper to taste

Instructions:

1. In a large bowl, combine salad greens, cherry tomatoes, cucumber, and red onion.

2. Top the salad with grilled chicken slices and diced avocado.

3. In a small bowl, whisk together olive oil and balsamic vinegar to create the dressing.

4. Drizzle the dressing over the salad.

5. Toss gently to coat the salad ingredients evenly.

6. Season with salt and pepper to taste.

7. Serve immediately for a fresh and satisfying low-carb lunch or dinner.

Nutritional Information (per serving):

- Calories: 450

- Protein: 30g

- Fat: 30g

- Carbohydrates: 12g

- Fiber: 6g

- Net Carbs: 6g

3. Zucchini Noodles with Pesto (All Phases)

Ingredients:

- 2 medium-sized zucchinis

- 1/4 cup basil pesto

- Cherry tomatoes, halved

- Grated Parmesan cheese (optional)

- Salt and pepper to taste

Instructions:

1. Using a spiralizer, create zucchini noodles.
2. Heat a skillet over medium heat and add the zucchini noodles.
3. Sauté for 2-3 minutes until the noodles are just tender.
4. Add basil pesto to the skillet and toss until the noodles are evenly coated.
5. Stir in cherry tomatoes and cook for an additional 1-2 minutes.
6. Season with salt and pepper to taste.
7. Optionally, sprinkle grated Parmesan cheese on top before serving.
8. This quick and flavorful zucchini noodle dish is a low-carb alternative to traditional pasta.

Nutritional Information (per serving):

- Calories: 180
- Protein: 5g
- Fat: 15g
- Carbohydrates: 8g
- Fiber: 3g
- Net Carbs: 5g

4. Baked Salmon with Lemon and Dill (All Phases)

Ingredients:

- 4 salmon fillets
- 1 lemon, thinly sliced

- Fresh dill, chopped
- 2 tbsp olive oil
- Salt and pepper to taste

Instructions:

1. Preheat the oven to 400°F (200°C).
2. Place salmon fillets on a baking sheet lined with parchment paper.
3. Drizzle olive oil over the salmon.
4. Season with salt and pepper.
5. Arrange lemon slices on top of each fillet and sprinkle with fresh dill.
6. Bake in the preheated oven for 12-15 minutes or until the salmon is cooked through.
7. Serve with a side of steamed vegetables for a light and flavorful low-carb dinner.

Nutritional Information (per serving):

- Calories: 350
- Protein: 30g
- Fat: 22g
- Carbohydrates: 2g
- Fiber: 1g
- Net Carbs: 1g

Ingredients:

- 1 cup mixed berries (strawberries, blueberries, raspberries)
- 1 cup Greek yogurt (unsweetened)
- 2 tbsp chopped nuts (almonds, walnuts)
- 1 tsp chia seeds (optional)
- 1 tsp honey (optional, for Balancing and beyond)

Instructions:

1. In a glass or bowl, layer Greek yogurt at the bottom.
2. Add a layer of mixed berries on top of the yogurt.
3. Repeat the layers until the glass is filled.
4. Sprinkle chopped nuts and chia seeds on the top layer.
5. Optionally, drizzle honey for added sweetness (if beyond the Induction Phase).
6. Enjoy this satisfying and nutrient-packed dessert or snack.

Nutritional Information (per serving):

- Calories: 250
- Protein: 15g
- Fat: 15g
- Carbohydrates: 20g
- Fiber: 6g
- Net Carbs: 14g

Ingredients:

- 1 large eggplant, thinly sliced lengthwise
- 1 lb ground beef or turkey
- 1 cup ricotta cheese
- 1 cup tomato sauce (sugar-free)
- 1 cup shredded mozzarella cheese
- Fresh basil, chopped
- Olive oil for cooking
- Salt and pepper to taste

Instructions:

1. Preheat the oven to 375°F (190°C).
2. In a skillet, brown the ground beef or turkey.
3. Season with salt and pepper and add tomato sauce to the meat.
4. In a separate pan, cook the eggplant slices in olive oil until softened.
5. In a baking dish, layer eggplant slices, meat sauce, ricotta cheese, and mozzarella cheese.
6. Repeat the layers until all ingredients are used.
7. Top the final layer with mozzarella cheese.
8. Bake in the preheated oven for 25-30 minutes or until the cheese is golden and bubbly.
9. Garnish with fresh basil before serving this delicious low-carb alternative to traditional lasagna.

Nutritional Information (per serving):

- Calories: 420
- Protein: 25g
- Fat: 30g
- Carbohydrates: 10g
- Fiber: 4g
- Net Carbs: 6g

7. Cauliflower Fried Rice (All Phases)

Ingredients:

- 1 head cauliflower, grated
- 2 cups mixed vegetables (peas, carrots, bell peppers), diced
- 2 eggs, beaten
- 3 tbsp soy sauce (or tamari for gluten-free)
- 2 tbsp sesame oil
- Green onions, chopped (for garnish)
- Salt and pepper to taste

Instructions:

1. In a food processor, pulse cauliflower until it reaches a rice-like consistency.
2. In a large skillet, heat sesame oil over medium heat.
3. Add mixed vegetables to the skillet and sauté until slightly tender.
4. Push the vegetables to one side of the skillet and pour beaten eggs into the empty side.

5. Scramble the eggs and incorporate them into the vegetables.

6. Add the cauliflower rice to the skillet.

7. Pour soy sauce over the mixture and stir until well combined.

8. Cook for an additional 5-7 minutes or until the cauliflower is tender.

9. Season with salt and pepper to taste.

10. Garnish with chopped green onions before serving this low-carb alternative to traditional fried rice.

Nutritional Information (per serving):

- Calories: 280

- Protein: 12g

- Fat: 20g

- Carbohydrates: 15g

- Fiber: 7g / Net Carbs: 8g

These beginner-friendly recipes cater to all phases of the Atkins Diet, offering a diverse range of flavors and textures to keep your meals exciting and satisfying. Experiment with these recipes, customize them to suit your preferences, and discover the delicious possibilities that the Atkins lifestyle has to offer—all while staying mindful of your nutritional goals.

Breakfast Recipes

1. Avocado and Bacon Breakfast Bowl

Ingredients:

- 1 ripe avocado, sliced
- 2 strips of cooked bacon, crumbled
- 2 large eggs, poached
- 1 tablespoon olive oil
- Salt and pepper to taste
- Optional: Chopped chives for garnish

Instructions:

1. In a bowl, arrange sliced avocado.
2. Top with poached eggs and crumbled bacon.
3. Drizzle with olive oil and season with salt and pepper.
4. Garnish with chopped chives if desired.

Nutritional Information:

- Calories: 450
- Protein: 20g
- Fat: 38g
- Carbohydrates: 10g
- Fiber: 7g

2. Spinach and Feta Omelette Roll

Ingredients:

- 3 large eggs, beaten

- 1 cup fresh spinach, chopped

- 1/4 cup feta cheese, crumbled

- 1 tablespoon olive oil

- Salt and pepper to taste

Instructions:

1. In a bowl, mix beaten eggs, chopped spinach, and crumbled feta.

2. Heat olive oil in a skillet over medium heat.

3. Pour the egg mixture into the skillet, spreading it evenly.

4. Cook until the edges set, then roll the omelette from one side to the other.

5. Season with salt and pepper.

Nutritional Information:

- Calories: 320

- Protein: 18g

- Fat: 25g

- Carbohydrates: 4g

- Fiber: 2g

3. Chia Seed Pudding with Berries

Ingredients:

- 2 tablespoons chia seeds

- 1/2 cup unsweetened almond milk

- 1/2 teaspoon vanilla extract

- 1/2 cup mixed berries (strawberries, blueberries, raspberries)

Instructions:

1. In a bowl, mix chia seeds, almond milk, and vanilla extract.

2. Let it sit in the refrigerator for at least 2 hours or overnight.

3. Before serving, top with mixed berries.

Nutritional Information:

- Calories: 180

- Protein: 5g

- Fat: 12g

- Carbohydrates: 15g

- Fiber: 8g

4. Greek Yogurt Parfait with Nuts and Seeds

Ingredients:

- 1 cup Greek yogurt

- 1/4 cup mixed nuts (almonds, walnuts) and seeds (sunflower, pumpkin)

- 1/2 teaspoon honey (optional)

- 1/4 teaspoon cinnamon

Instructions:

1. In a glass, layer Greek yogurt with mixed nuts and seeds.

2. Drizzle with honey if desired.

3. Sprinkle with cinnamon before serving.

Nutritional Information:

- Calories: 320
- Protein: 20g
- Fat: 18g
- Carbohydrates: 20g
- Fiber: 4g

5. Low-Carb Breakfast Burrito Bowl

Ingredients:

- 2 large eggs, scrambled
- 1/4 cup shredded cheddar cheese
- 1/2 cup cauliflower rice, cooked
- 1/4 cup salsa
- 1/4 avocado, sliced

Instructions:

1. In a bowl, layer cauliflower rice, scrambled eggs, and shredded cheese.
2. Top with salsa and sliced avocado.

Nutritional Information:

- Calories: 380
- Protein: 22g
- Fat: 28g
- Carbohydrates: 10g
- Fiber: 5g

Adjust portion sizes based on individual dietary needs and preferences.

Variety for Every Palate

1. Zucchini and Cheese Breakfast Muffins

Ingredients:

- 2 medium-sized zucchinis, grated
- 4 eggs, beaten
- 1 cup shredded cheddar cheese
- 1/4 cup almond flour
- 1 teaspoon baking powder
- Salt and pepper to taste

Instructions:

1. Preheat the oven to 375°F (190°C).
2. In a bowl, mix grated zucchini, beaten eggs, cheddar cheese, almond flour, baking powder, salt, and pepper.
3. Spoon the mixture into muffin cups.
4. Bake for 20-25 minutes or until the muffins are golden brown.

Nutritional Information:

- Calories: 180
- Protein: 12g
- Fat: 14g
- Carbohydrates: 4g
- Fiber: 1g

Ingredients:

- 2 bell peppers, halved and seeds removed
- 4 oz smoked salmon
- 1/2 cup cream cheese, softened
- Chives for garnish

Instructions:

1. Preheat the oven to 350°F (175°C).
2. In a bowl, mix smoked salmon and softened cream cheese.
3. Stuff the bell pepper halves with the mixture.
4. Bake for 15-20 minutes or until the peppers are tender.
5. Garnish with chives before serving.

Nutritional Information:

- Calories: 250
- Protein: 15g
- Fat: 18g
- Carbohydrates: 7g
- Fiber: 2g

3. Coconut Flour Pancakes with Berries

Ingredients:

- 1/4 cup coconut flour
- 4 eggs
- 1/2 cup unsweetened almond milk
- 1 teaspoon baking powder
- Mixed berries for topping

Instructions:

1. In a bowl, whisk coconut flour, eggs, almond milk, and baking powder.
2. Heat a griddle or skillet over medium heat.
3. Spoon the batter onto the griddle to make pancakes.
4. Cook until bubbles form, then flip and cook the other side.
5. Top with mixed berries before serving.

Nutritional Information:

- Calories: 220
- Protein: 12g
- Fat: 14g
- Carbohydrates: 10g
- Fiber: 6g

Ingredients:

- 2 cups cauliflower rice
- 1 egg, beaten
- 1/4 cup grated parmesan cheese
- 1/2 teaspoon garlic powder
- Salt and pepper to taste
- Avocado salsa for topping

Instructions:

1. Preheat the oven to 400°F (200°C).
2. In a bowl, mix cauliflower rice, beaten egg, parmesan cheese, garlic powder, salt, and pepper.
3. Form the mixture into hash brown patties on a baking sheet.
4. Bake for 20-25 minutes or until golden brown.
5. Top with avocado salsa before serving.

Nutritional Information:

- Calories: 180
- Protein: 10g
- Fat: 12g
- Carbohydrates: 10g
- Fiber: 4g

Ingredients:

- 1/2 lb ground turkey
- 1 bell pepper, diced
- 1 zucchini, diced
- 4 eggs
- 1 tablespoon olive oil
- Salt and pepper to taste

Instructions:

1. In a skillet, brown ground turkey in olive oil.
2. Add diced bell pepper and zucchini, cooking until vegetables are tender.
3. Make wells in the mixture and crack eggs into them.
4. Cover and cook until the eggs are done to your liking.
5. Season with salt and pepper before serving.

Nutritional Information:

- Calories: 340
- Protein: 25g
- Fat: 22g
- Carbohydrates: 10g
- Fiber: 3g

Adjust portion sizes based on individual dietary needs and preferences.

LUNCH RECIPES

Nutrient-Packed Midday Fuel

1. Grilled Chicken Salad with Avocado Dressing

Ingredients:

- 6 oz grilled chicken breast, sliced
- Mixed salad greens (spinach, arugula, and kale)
- 1 avocado, mashed
- 2 tablespoons olive oil
- 1 tablespoon lemon juice
- Salt and pepper to taste

Instructions:

1. Arrange the mixed salad greens on a plate.
2. Top with sliced grilled chicken.
3. In a bowl, whisk together mashed avocado, olive oil, lemon juice, salt, and pepper to make the dressing.
4. Drizzle the avocado dressing over the salad before serving.

Nutritional Information:

- Calories: 420
- Protein: 30g
- Fat: 28g
- Carbohydrates: 10g
- Fiber: 7g

2. Egg Salad Lettuce Wraps

Ingredients:

- 4 hard-boiled eggs, chopped
- 1/4 cup mayonnaise
- 1 teaspoon Dijon mustard
- 1/2 cup celery, finely chopped
- Lettuce leaves for wrapping

Instructions:

1. In a bowl, mix chopped hard-boiled eggs, mayonnaise, Dijon mustard, and chopped celery.
2. Spoon the egg salad onto lettuce leaves.
3. Roll the leaves to create wraps.

Nutritional Information:

- Calories: 320
- Protein: 16g
- Fat: 28g
- Carbohydrates: 2g
- Fiber: 1g

3. Salmon and Avocado Nori Rolls

Ingredients:

- Nori seaweed sheets
- 4 oz smoked salmon
- 1 avocado, sliced
- Cucumber strips
- 1 tablespoon soy sauce (low sodium)

Instructions:

1. Lay a nori sheet on a flat surface.

2. Arrange smoked salmon, avocado slices, and cucumber strips.

3. Roll tightly and slice into bite-sized pieces.

4. Serve with a side of low-sodium soy sauce.

Nutritional Information:

- Calories: 280

- Protein: 20g

- Fat: 18g

- Carbohydrates: 8g

- Fiber: 5g

4. Turkey and Vegetable Lettuce Wraps

Ingredients:

- 1/2 lb ground turkey

- 1 tablespoon olive oil

- 1 bell pepper, diced

- 1 zucchini, diced

- Lettuce leaves for wrapping

- 1/4 cup shredded cheddar cheese

Instructions:

1. In a skillet, brown ground turkey in olive oil.

2. Add diced bell pepper and zucchini, cooking until vegetables are tender.

3. Spoon the turkey and vegetable mixture onto lettuce leaves.

4. Top with shredded cheddar cheese.

Nutritional Information:

- Calories: 350
- Protein: 24g
- Fat: 22g
- Carbohydrates: 10g
- Fiber: 4g

5. Cauliflower and Broccoli Salad with Feta

Ingredients:

- 2 cups cauliflower florets, steamed
- 2 cups broccoli florets, steamed
- 1/4 cup red onion, finely chopped
- 1/4 cup feta cheese, crumbled
- 2 tablespoons olive oil
- 1 tablespoon balsamic vinegar
- Salt and pepper to taste

Instructions:

1. In a bowl, combine steamed cauliflower and broccoli.
2. Add chopped red onion and crumbled feta.
3. In a small bowl, whisk together olive oil and balsamic vinegar.
4. Drizzle the dressing over the salad and toss.
5. Season with salt and pepper before serving.

Nutritional Information:

- Calories: 280
- Protein: 10g
- Fat: 22g
- Carbohydrates: 14g
- Fiber: 6g

Adjust portion sizes based on individual dietary needs and preferences.

Quick and Satisfying Options

1. Shrimp and Avocado Lettuce Wraps

Ingredients:

- 1/2 lb shrimp, cooked and peeled
- 1 avocado, sliced
- Lettuce leaves for wrapping
- 1 tablespoon olive oil
- Lime wedges for serving

Instructions:

1. In a skillet, heat olive oil and sauté cooked shrimp briefly.
2. Spoon shrimp and sliced avocado onto lettuce leaves.
3. Squeeze lime juice over the wraps before serving.

Nutritional Information:

- Calories: 300

- Protein: 20g

- Fat: 18g

- Carbohydrates: 10g

- Fiber: 6g

2. Caprese Chicken Salad Bowl

Ingredients:

- 6 oz grilled chicken breast, sliced

- 1 cup cherry tomatoes, halved

- 1/2 cup fresh mozzarella balls

- Fresh basil leaves

- Balsamic vinaigrette dressing

Instructions:

1. Arrange sliced grilled chicken, cherry tomatoes, and mozzarella balls in a bowl.

2. Garnish with fresh basil leaves.

3. Drizzle with balsamic vinaigrette dressing before serving.

Nutritional Information:

- Calories: 380

- Protein: 30g

- Fat: 22g

- Carbohydrates: 8g

- Fiber: 2g

3. Turkey and Spinach Stuffed Mushrooms

Ingredients:

- 1/2 lb ground turkey
- 8 large mushrooms, stems removed
- 1 cup spinach, chopped
- 1/4 cup feta cheese, crumbled
- 1 tablespoon olive oil

Instructions:

1. Preheat the oven to 375°F (190°C).
2. In a skillet, brown ground turkey in olive oil.
3. Mix in chopped spinach and crumbled feta.
4. Stuff mushrooms with the turkey and spinach mixture.
5. Bake for 15-20 minutes or until mushrooms are tender.

Nutritional Information:

- Calories: 290
- Protein: 25g
- Fat: 18g
- Carbohydrates: 6g
- Fiber: 2g

Ingredients:

- 6 oz grilled chicken breast, sliced
- 2 hard-boiled eggs, sliced
- 4 slices bacon, cooked and crumbled
- 1/2 avocado, sliced
- Lettuce leaves for wrapping

Instructions:

1. Lay out lettuce leaves and evenly distribute chicken, eggs, bacon, and avocado.
2. Roll the leaves to create wraps.

Nutritional Information:

- Calories: 420
- Protein: 30g
- Fat: 28g
- Carbohydrates: 8g
- Fiber: 4g

5. Mediterranean Tuna Salad

Ingredients:

- 1 can tuna, drained
- 1/4 cup Kalamata olives, sliced
- 1/4 cup cherry tomatoes, halved
- 1/4 cup cucumber, diced
- Feta cheese, crumbled
- Olive oil and lemon juice dressing

Instructions:

1. In a bowl, combine drained tuna, olives, cherry tomatoes, and diced cucumber.

2. Drizzle with olive oil and lemon juice dressing.

3. Top with crumbled feta cheese before serving.

Nutritional Information:

- Calories: 320

- Protein: 25g

- Fat: 22g

- Carbohydrates: 6g

- Fiber: 2g

Adjust portion sizes based on individual dietary needs and preferences.

DINNER RECIPES

1. Grilled Salmon with Lemon Dill Sauce

Ingredients:

- 1 lb salmon fillets
- 1 tablespoon olive oil
- Salt and pepper to taste
- 1 lemon, juiced
- 2 tablespoons fresh dill, chopped

Instructions:

1. Preheat the grill to medium-high heat.
2. Brush salmon fillets with olive oil and season with salt and pepper.
3. Grill for 4-5 minutes per side or until cooked through.
4. In a bowl, mix lemon juice and chopped dill to create the sauce.
5. Drizzle the sauce over the grilled salmon before serving.

Nutritional Information:

- Calories: 380
- Protein: 35g
- Fat: 25g
- Carbohydrates: 2g
- Fiber: 0.5g

Ingredients:

- 1 cauliflower pizza crust
- 1/2 cup sugar-free pizza sauce
- 1 cup shredded mozzarella cheese
- Assorted vegetables (bell peppers, mushrooms, onions)

Instructions:

1. Preheat the oven according to the cauliflower crust package instructions.
2. Spread pizza sauce over the crust.
3. Sprinkle shredded mozzarella cheese and add chopped vegetables.
4. Bake as directed until the crust is golden and cheese is melted.

Nutritional Information:

- Calories: 280
- Protein: 20g
- Fat: 18g
- Carbohydrates: 12g
- Fiber: 6g

Ingredients:

- 2 medium zucchinis, spiralized
- 4 slices bacon, chopped
- 3 eggs
- 1/2 cup grated Parmesan cheese
- Salt and black pepper to taste

Instructions:

1. In a skillet, cook chopped bacon until crispy.
2. Whisk together eggs and Parmesan cheese in a bowl.
3. Add spiralized zucchini to the skillet and cook until tender.
4. Pour the egg and cheese mixture over the zoodles, stirring quickly.
5. Season with salt and pepper before serving.

Nutritional Information:

- Calories: 320
- Protein: 18g
- Fat: 22g
- Carbohydrates: 10g
- Fiber: 3g

4. Grilled Chicken Caesar Salad

Ingredients:

- 6 oz grilled chicken breast, sliced
- Romaine lettuce, chopped
- 1/4 cup grated Parmesan cheese
- Caesar dressing (low-carb)

Instructions:

1. Grill chicken until cooked through and slice into strips.
2. In a large bowl, toss chopped romaine with sliced chicken.
3. Sprinkle grated Parmesan over the salad.
4. Drizzle with Caesar dressing before serving.

Nutritional Information:

- Calories: 340
- Protein: 28g
- Fat: 22g
- Carbohydrates: 6g
- Fiber: 3g

5. Eggplant Lasagna with Ground Beef

Ingredients:

- 1 large eggplant, sliced
- 1 lb ground beef
- 1 cup sugar-free marinara sauce
- 1 cup ricotta cheese
- 1 cup shredded mozzarella cheese
- Italian seasoning, salt, and pepper to taste

Instructions:

1. Preheat the oven to 375°F (190°C).
2. In a skillet, brown ground beef and season with Italian seasoning, salt, and pepper.
3. In a baking dish, layer sliced eggplant, ground beef, ricotta, and marinara sauce.
4. Repeat the layers and top with shredded mozzarella.
5. Bake for 30-35 minutes or until bubbly and golden.

Nutritional Information:

- Calories: 420
- Protein: 30g
- Fat: 28g
- Carbohydrates: 10g
- Fiber: 4g

Adjust portion sizes based on individual dietary needs and preferences.

Wholesome and Flavorful Choices

Ingredients:

- 4 bell peppers, halved and seeds removed
- 1 lb ground turkey
- 1 cup cauliflower rice
- 1/2 cup diced tomatoes
- 1/4 cup chopped onions
- 1 teaspoon garlic powder
- 1 teaspoon Italian seasoning
- Salt and pepper to taste
- 1/2 cup shredded cheddar cheese (optional)

Instructions:

1. Preheat the oven to 375°F (190°C).
2. In a skillet, cook ground turkey until browned.
3. Add cauliflower rice, diced tomatoes, onions, garlic powder, Italian seasoning, salt, and pepper. Cook until vegetables are tender.
4. Stuff the bell peppers with the turkey and cauliflower rice mixture.
5. Optional: Top with shredded cheddar cheese.
6. Bake for 25-30 minutes or until peppers are tender.

Nutritional Information:

- Calories: 320
- Protein: 28g
- Fat: 18g
- Carbohydrates: 10g
- Fiber: 3g

2. Garlic Butter Shrimp with Zucchini Noodles

Ingredients:

- 1 lb shrimp, peeled and deveined
- 4 medium zucchinis, spiralized
- 3 tablespoons unsalted butter
- 4 cloves garlic, minced
- 1/4 cup chopped parsley
- Salt and pepper to taste
- Red pepper flakes (optional)

Instructions:

1. In a skillet, melt butter over medium heat.
2. Add minced garlic and sauté until fragrant.
3. Add shrimp and cook until pink.
4. Toss in spiralized zucchini and cook until tender.
5. Season with salt, pepper, and red pepper flakes if desired.
6. Garnish with chopped parsley before serving.

Nutritional Information:

- Calories: 280
- Protein: 24g
- Fat: 18g
- Carbohydrates: 8g
- Fiber: 2g

3. Spaghetti Squash Bolognese

Ingredients:

- 1 medium spaghetti squash, halved and seeds removed
- 1 lb ground beef
- 1 cup sugar-free marinara sauce
- 1/2 cup diced onions
- 2 cloves garlic, minced
- 1 teaspoon dried oregano
- Salt and pepper to taste
- Fresh basil for garnish

Instructions:

1. Preheat the oven to 375°F (190°C).
2. Roast spaghetti squash halves in the oven until fork-tender.
3. In a skillet, brown ground beef with onions and garlic.
4. Stir in marinara sauce and oregano, simmering until heated through.
5. Scrape the spaghetti squash with a fork to create "noodles."

6. Serve the bolognese sauce over the spaghetti squash.

7. Garnish with fresh basil before serving.

Nutritional Information:

- Calories: 350
- Protein: 28g
- Fat: 20g
- Carbohydrates: 12g
- Fiber: 4g

4. Baked Chicken Thighs with Rosemary and Lemon

Ingredients:

- 4 bone-in, skin-on chicken thighs
- 2 tablespoons olive oil
- 1 tablespoon fresh rosemary, chopped
- 2 cloves garlic, minced
- Zest and juice of 1 lemon
- Salt and pepper to taste

Instructions:

1. Preheat the oven to 400°F (200°C).

2. In a bowl, mix olive oil, rosemary, minced garlic, lemon zest, and lemon juice.

3. Place chicken thighs in a baking dish and rub the mixture over them.

4. Season with salt and pepper.

5. Bake for 35-40 minutes or until chicken is golden and cooked through.

Nutritional Information:

- Calories: 380
- Protein: 32g
- Fat: 28g
- Carbohydrates: 1g
- Fiber: 0.5g

5. Eggplant Parmesan

Ingredients:

- 1 large eggplant, sliced
- 2 eggs, beaten
- 1 cup almond flour
- 1 cup sugar-free marinara sauce
- 1 cup shredded mozzarella cheese
- 1/2 cup grated Parmesan cheese
- Fresh basil for garnish

Instructions:

1. Preheat the oven to 375°F (190°C).
2. Dip eggplant slices in beaten eggs, then coat with almond flour.
3. Bake on a parchment-lined baking sheet until golden.
4. In a baking dish, layer baked eggplant slices, marinara sauce, and cheeses.
5. Repeat the layers and bake for 25-30 minutes.
6. Garnish with fresh basil before serving.

Nutritional Information:

- Calories: 320
- Protein: 16g
- Fat: 24g
- Carbohydrates: 12g
- Fiber: 5g

Adjust portion sizes based on individual dietary needs and preferences.

SNACK RECIPES

1. Parmesan and Rosemary Almond Crackers

Ingredients:

- 1 cup almond flour
- 1 cup grated Parmesan cheese
- 1 tablespoon fresh rosemary, finely chopped
- 1 egg
- 1/2 teaspoon garlic powder
- Salt to taste

Instructions:

1. Preheat the oven to 350°F (175°C).
2. In a bowl, combine almond flour, Parmesan cheese, rosemary, garlic powder, and salt.
3. Add the egg and mix until a dough forms.
4. Roll out the dough between two sheets of parchment paper.
5. Cut into squares or use cookie cutters.
6. Transfer to a baking sheet and bake for 12-15 minutes or until golden.

Nutritional Information:

- Calories: 120
- Protein: 7g
- Fat: 9g
- Carbohydrates: 3g
- Fiber: 1g

2. Cucumber and Cream Cheese Bites

Ingredients:

- 1 cucumber, sliced
- 4 oz cream cheese, softened
- Smoked salmon (optional)
- Fresh dill for garnish

Instructions:

1. Spread cream cheese on cucumber slices.
2. Top with smoked salmon if desired.
3. Garnish with fresh dill.

Nutritional Information:

- Calories: 100
- Protein: 3g
- Fat: 9g
- Carbohydrates: 2g
- Fiber: 0.5g

3. Avocado and Bacon Deviled Eggs

Ingredients:

- 6 hard-boiled eggs, halved
- 1 ripe avocado, mashed
- 2 slices bacon, cooked and crumbled
- 1 tablespoon mayonnaise
- Salt and pepper to taste
- Paprika for garnish

Instructions:

1. Remove egg yolks and mash with avocado, bacon, and mayonnaise.

2. Season with salt and pepper.

3. Spoon the mixture back into egg whites.

4. Garnish with paprika.

Nutritional Information:

- Calories: 180

- Protein: 9g

- Fat: 15g

- Carbohydrates: 3g

- Fiber: 2g

4. Spicy Roasted Chickpeas

Ingredients:

- 1 can (15 oz) chickpeas, drained and rinsed

- 1 tablespoon olive oil

- 1 teaspoon smoked paprika

- 1/2 teaspoon cayenne pepper

- Salt to taste

Instructions:

1. Preheat the oven to 400°F (200°C).

2. Pat chickpeas dry and toss with olive oil, smoked paprika, cayenne pepper, and salt.

3. Spread on a baking sheet and roast for 25-30 minutes or until crispy.

Nutritional Information:

- Calories: 160
- Protein: 6g
- Fat: 6g
- Carbohydrates: 22g
- Fiber: 6g

5. Dark Chocolate and Almond Clusters

Ingredients:

- 1/2 cup dark chocolate chips (70% cocoa or higher)
- 1/2 cup almonds, chopped
- Sea salt for sprinkling

Instructions:

1. Melt dark chocolate chips in a heatproof bowl.
2. Stir in chopped almonds.
3. Drop spoonfuls onto a parchment-lined tray.
4. Sprinkle with sea salt and refrigerate until set.

Nutritional Information:

- Calories: 180
- Protein: 5g
- Fat: 14g
- Carbohydrates: 12g
- Fiber: 4g

Adjust portion sizes based on individual dietary needs and preferences.

Satisfying Cravings Smartly

1. Guacamole Stuffed Cucumber Bites

Ingredients:

- 2 cucumbers, sliced into rounds
- 2 ripe avocados, mashed
- 1 tablespoon lime juice
- 1/4 cup cherry tomatoes, diced
- 1 tablespoon red onion, finely chopped
- Salt and pepper to taste
- Fresh cilantro for garnish

Instructions:

1. In a bowl, mix mashed avocados, lime juice, diced cherry tomatoes, red onion, salt, and pepper.
2. Scoop out a small portion of each cucumber round to create a cup.
3. Spoon guacamole into the cucumber cups.
4. Garnish with fresh cilantro before serving.

Nutritional Information:

- Calories: 150
- Protein: 2g
- Fat: 13g
- Carbohydrates: 9g
- Fiber: 6g

2. Protein-Packed Greek Yogurt Parfait

Ingredients:

- 1 cup plain Greek yogurt

- 1/2 cup mixed berries (strawberries, blueberries, raspberries)

- 1/4 cup chopped nuts (almonds, walnuts)

- 1 tablespoon chia seeds

- 1 teaspoon honey (optional)

Instructions:

1. In a glass, layer Greek yogurt with mixed berries, chopped nuts, and chia seeds.

2. Drizzle with honey if desired.

3. Repeat layers and serve chilled.

Nutritional Information:

- Calories: 250

- Protein: 18g

- Fat: 15g

- Carbohydrates: 15g

- Fiber: 6g

3. Cheese and Pepperoni Roll-Ups

Ingredients:

- 8 slices pepperoni

- 4 slices mozzarella cheese

- 1 tablespoon cream cheese

- Fresh basil leaves

Instructions:

1. Spread a thin layer of cream cheese on each mozzarella slice.

2. Place 2 slices of pepperoni on each cheese slice.

3. Add a basil leaf to each and roll up.

4. Secure with toothpicks and serve.

Nutritional Information:

- Calories: 200

- Protein: 12g

- Fat: 16g

- Carbohydrates: 1g

- Fiber: 0g

4. Spicy Buffalo Cauliflower Bites

Ingredients:

- 2 cups cauliflower florets

- 2 tablespoons olive oil

- 1/4 cup buffalo sauce

- 1/2 teaspoon garlic powder

- Celery sticks for serving

- Ranch dressing for dipping

Instructions:

1. Preheat the oven to 450°F (230°C).

2. Toss cauliflower florets with olive oil and garlic powder.

3. Roast for 20 minutes, then toss in buffalo sauce.

4. Roast for an additional 10-15 minutes until crispy.

5. Serve with celery sticks and ranch dressing.

Nutritional Information:

- Calories: 180
- Protein: 4g
- Fat: 14g
- Carbohydrates: 8g
- Fiber: 3g

5. Chocolate Avocado Mousse

Ingredients:

- 2 ripe avocados
- 1/4 cup unsweetened cocoa powder
- 1/4 cup almond milk
- 1/4 cup powdered erythritol (or sweetener of choice)
- 1 teaspoon vanilla extract

Instructions:

1. Blend avocados, cocoa powder, almond milk, erythritol, and vanilla extract until smooth.
2. Chill in the refrigerator for at least 1 hour.
3. Serve in small bowls or cups.

Nutritional Information:

- Calories: 220
- Protein: 4g
- Fat: 18g
- Carbohydrates: 14g
- Fiber: 9g

Adjust portion sizes based on individual dietary needs and preferences.

SOUP AND SALAD RECIPES

1. Chicken and Vegetable Zoodle Soup

Ingredients:

- 1 lb chicken breasts, cooked and shredded
- 4 cups chicken broth (low sodium)
- 2 zucchinis, spiralized
- 1 cup celery, diced
- 1 cup carrots, julienned
- 1 cup kale, chopped
- 2 cloves garlic, minced
- 1 teaspoon thyme
- Salt and pepper to taste

Instructions:

1. In a pot, bring chicken broth to a simmer.
2. Add shredded chicken, spiralized zucchini, celery, carrots, kale, garlic, thyme, salt, and pepper.
3. Simmer for 15-20 minutes until vegetables are tender.
4. Adjust seasoning if needed before serving.

Nutritional Information:

- Calories: 180
- Protein: 25g
- Fat: 4g
- Carbohydrates: 10g / Fiber: 3g

Ingredients:

- 1 lb shrimp, cooked and peeled
- 2 avocados, diced
- 1 cup cherry tomatoes, halved
- 1/4 cup red onion, finely chopped
- Mixed salad greens
- 2 tablespoons olive oil
- 1 tablespoon lemon juice
- Salt and pepper to taste

Instructions:

1. In a bowl, combine cooked shrimp, diced avocados, cherry tomatoes, red onion, and mixed salad greens.
2. In a small bowl, whisk together olive oil, lemon juice, salt, and pepper to create the dressing.
3. Drizzle the dressing over the salad before serving.

Nutritional Information:

- Calories: 320
- Protein: 20g
- Fat: 24g
- Carbohydrates: 14g
- Fiber: 8g

3. Creamy Broccoli and Cheddar Soup

Ingredients:

- 4 cups broccoli florets
- 1/2 cup onion, chopped
- 2 cloves garlic, minced
- 4 cups chicken broth (low sodium)
- 1 cup cheddar cheese, shredded
- 1/2 cup heavy cream
- Salt and pepper to taste

Instructions:

1. In a pot, sauté chopped onion and minced garlic until softened.
2. Add broccoli florets and chicken broth, bringing to a simmer.
3. Cook until broccoli is tender, then blend until smooth.
4. Stir in shredded cheddar cheese and heavy cream.
5. Season with salt and pepper before serving.

Nutritional Information:

- Calories: 250
- Protein: 12g
- Fat: 20g
- Carbohydrates: 10g
- Fiber: 4g

Ingredients:

- 6 oz grilled turkey breast, sliced
- Mixed salad greens
- 2 hard-boiled eggs, sliced
- 1 avocado, diced
- 4 slices bacon, cooked and crumbled
- 1/4 cup blue cheese, crumbled
- Ranch dressing (low-carb)

Instructions:

1. Arrange mixed salad greens on a plate.
2. Top with grilled turkey, sliced hard-boiled eggs, diced avocado, crumbled bacon, and blue cheese.
3. Drizzle with ranch dressing before serving.

Nutritional Information:

- Calories: 380
- Protein: 30g
- Fat: 28g
- Carbohydrates: 8g
- Fiber: 4g

Ingredients:

- 4 cups spinach, chopped
- 1 cup mushrooms, sliced
- 1/2 cup onion, chopped
- 2 cloves garlic, minced
- 4 cups vegetable broth (low sodium)
- 1/2 cup heavy cream
- 2 tablespoons olive oil
- Salt and pepper to taste

Instructions:

1. In a pot, sauté chopped onion and minced garlic in olive oil until softened.
2. Add sliced mushrooms and cook until tender.
3. Pour in vegetable broth and bring to a simmer.
4. Stir in chopped spinach and heavy cream.
5. Season with salt and pepper before serving.

Nutritional Information:

- Calories: 220
- Protein: 6g
- Fat: 18g
- Carbohydrates: 10g
- Fiber: 4g

Adjust portion sizes based on individual dietary needs and preferences.

CREATIVE AND FILLING CREATIONS

Low-Carb Twists on Classics

1. Cauliflower Crust Margherita Pizza

Ingredients:

- 1 medium-sized cauliflower, grated
- 1 cup mozzarella cheese, shredded
- 1 egg
- 1 teaspoon dried oregano
- 1/2 cup sugar-free pizza sauce
- Fresh basil leaves
- Cherry tomatoes, sliced

Instructions:

1. Preheat the oven to 425°F (220°C).
2. Mix grated cauliflower, shredded mozzarella, egg, and oregano in a bowl.
3. Press the mixture onto a parchment-lined baking sheet to form a crust.
4. Bake for 15-20 minutes until golden.
5. Spread sugar-free pizza sauce on the crust and top with fresh basil and sliced cherry tomatoes.
6. Bake for an additional 10 minutes.

Nutritional Information:

- Calories: 180
- Protein: 12g
- Fat: 10g

- Carbohydrates: 8g

- Fiber: 3g

2. Zucchini Noodles with Pesto and Cherry Tomatoes

Ingredients:

- 2 medium zucchinis, spiralized

- 1 cup cherry tomatoes, halved

- 1/4 cup pine nuts

- 1/2 cup fresh basil leaves

- 1/4 cup grated Parmesan cheese

- 2 cloves garlic

- 1/3 cup olive oil

- Salt and pepper to taste

Instructions:

1. In a food processor, blend pine nuts, basil, Parmesan, and garlic.

2. With the processor running, slowly add olive oil until smooth.

3. Toss spiralized zucchini with pesto and cherry tomatoes.

4. Season with salt and pepper before serving.

Nutritional Information:

- Calories: 220

- Protein: 5g

- Fat: 20g

- Carbohydrates: 6g

- Fiber: 2g

Ingredients:

- 1 large eggplant, sliced
- 1 lb ground turkey
- 1 cup sugar-free marinara sauce
- 1 cup ricotta cheese
- 1 cup shredded mozzarella cheese
- Italian seasoning, salt, and pepper to taste

Instructions:

1. Preheat the oven to 375°F (190°C).
2. In a skillet, brown ground turkey and season with Italian seasoning, salt, and pepper.
3. In a baking dish, layer sliced eggplant, ground turkey, ricotta, and marinara sauce.
4. Repeat the layers and top with shredded mozzarella.
5. Bake for 30-35 minutes or until bubbly and golden.

Nutritional Information:

- Calories: 380
- Protein: 30g
- Fat: 22g
- Carbohydrates: 10g
- Fiber: 4g

Ingredients:

- 4 cabbage leaves, blanched
- 1 lb chicken breast, cooked and shredded
- 1/2 cup diced bell peppers
- 1/4 cup diced onions
- 1 cup enchilada sauce (sugar-free)
- 1 cup shredded cheddar cheese
- Fresh cilantro for garnish

Instructions:

1. Mix shredded chicken, diced bell peppers, and onions in a bowl.
2. Place a portion of the mixture onto each cabbage leaf.
3. Roll up the leaves and place them seam side down in a baking dish.
4. Pour enchilada sauce over the cabbage rolls and top with shredded cheddar.
5. Bake for 20-25 minutes until cheese is melted and bubbly.
6. Garnish with fresh cilantro before serving.

Nutritional Information:

- Calories: 320
- Protein: 28g
- Fat: 18g
- Carbohydrates: 8g / Fiber: 3g

5. Low-Carb Broccoli Cheddar Soup

Ingredients:

- 2 cups broccoli florets
- 1/2 cup onion, chopped
- 2 cloves garlic, minced
- 4 cups chicken broth (low sodium)
- 1 cup cheddar cheese, shredded
- 1/2 cup heavy cream
- 2 tablespoons olive oil
- Salt and pepper to taste

Instructions:

1. In a pot, sauté chopped onion and minced garlic in olive oil until softened.
2. Add broccoli florets and chicken broth, bringing to a simmer.
3. Cook until broccoli is tender, then blend until smooth.
4. Stir in shredded cheddar cheese and heavy cream.
5. Season with salt and pepper before serving.

Nutritional Information:

- Calories: 250
- Protein: 12g
- Fat: 20g
- Carbohydrates: 8g
- Fiber: 3g

Adjust portion sizes based on individual dietary needs and preferences.

Meat and Seafood Recipes

1. Grilled Lemon Garlic Shrimp Skewers

Ingredients:

- 1 lb large shrimp, peeled and deveined
- 2 tablespoons olive oil
- 2 cloves garlic, minced
- Zest of one lemon
- 1 tablespoon fresh lemon juice
- 1 teaspoon dried oregano
- Salt and pepper to taste

Instructions:

1. In a bowl, mix olive oil, minced garlic, lemon zest, lemon juice, oregano, salt, and pepper.
2. Thread shrimp onto skewers and brush with the marinade.
3. Grill for 2-3 minutes per side until opaque and lightly charred.
4. Serve immediately.

Nutritional Information:

- Calories: 180
- Protein: 25g
- Fat: 9g
- Carbohydrates: 2g
- Fiber: 0g

2. Baked Parmesan Crusted Chicken Tenders

Ingredients:

- 1 lb chicken tenders
- 1 cup almond flour
- 1/2 cup grated Parmesan cheese
- 1 teaspoon garlic powder
- 1 teaspoon paprika
- 2 eggs, beaten
- Salt and pepper to taste

Instructions:

1. Preheat the oven to 400°F (200°C).
2. In a bowl, mix almond flour, grated Parmesan, garlic powder, paprika, salt, and pepper.
3. Dip each chicken tender into beaten eggs, then coat with the almond flour mixture.
4. Place on a baking sheet and bake for 15-20 minutes until golden and cooked through.
5. Serve with a low-carb dipping sauce.

Nutritional Information:

- Calories: 280
- Protein: 30g
- Fat: 16g
- Carbohydrates: 4g
- Fiber: 2g

3. Lemon Herb Baked Salmon

Ingredients:

- 4 salmon fillets
- 2 tablespoons olive oil
- Zest of one lemon
- 2 tablespoons fresh lemon juice
- 1 teaspoon dried thyme
- 1 teaspoon dried rosemary
- Salt and pepper to taste

Instructions:

1. Preheat the oven to 375°F (190°C).
2. In a bowl, mix olive oil, lemon zest, lemon juice, thyme, rosemary, salt, and pepper.
3. Place salmon fillets on a baking sheet and brush with the lemon herb mixture.
4. Bake for 15-20 minutes until salmon flakes easily with a fork.
5. Garnish with fresh herbs before serving.

Nutritional Information:

- Calories: 300
- Protein: 25g
- Fat: 20g
- Carbohydrates: 1g
- Fiber: 0g

Ingredients:

- 1 lb ground turkey
- 1 cup grated zucchini, squeezed dry
- 1/4 cup almond flour
- 1/4 cup grated Parmesan cheese
- 1 teaspoon dried basil
- 1 teaspoon dried oregano
- 1/2 teaspoon garlic powder
- Salt and pepper to taste

Instructions:

1. Preheat the oven to 400°F (200°C).
2. In a bowl, mix ground turkey, grated zucchini, almond flour, grated Parmesan, basil, oregano, garlic powder, salt, and pepper.
3. Form into meatballs and place on a baking sheet.
4. Bake for 20-25 minutes until cooked through and golden.
5. Serve with a low-carb marinara sauce.

Nutritional Information:

- Calories: 220
- Protein: 28g
- Fat: 10g
- Carbohydrates: 3g
- Fiber: 1g

Ingredients:

- 1 lb sirloin or ribeye steak, cut into bite-sized pieces
- 3 tablespoons unsalted butter
- 3 cloves garlic, minced
- 1 teaspoon dried thyme
- Salt and pepper to taste
- Fresh parsley for garnish

Instructions:

1. In a skillet, melt butter over medium heat.
2. Add minced garlic and cook until fragrant.
3. Add steak bites, thyme, salt, and pepper.
4. Cook for 3-4 minutes per side until browned.
5. Garnish with fresh parsley before serving.

Nutritional Information:

- Calories: 340
- Protein: 30g
- Fat: 22g
- Carbohydrates: 1g
- Fiber: 0g

Adjust portion sizes based on individual dietary needs and preferences.

PROTEIN-PACKED DELIGHTS

Seafood Sensations

1. Lemon Garlic Butter Shrimp Scampi

Ingredients:

- 1 lb large shrimp, peeled and deveined
- 3 tablespoons unsalted butter
- 3 cloves garlic, minced
- Zest of one lemon
- 2 tablespoons fresh lemon juice
- 1/4 cup fresh parsley, chopped
- Salt and pepper to taste

Instructions:

1. In a skillet, melt butter over medium heat.
2. Add minced garlic and sauté until fragrant.
3. Add shrimp, lemon zest, and lemon juice.
4. Cook for 2-3 minutes per side until shrimp are opaque.
5. Season with salt and pepper, sprinkle with fresh parsley, and serve.

Nutritional Information:

- Calories: 220
- Protein: 25g
- Fat: 13g
- Carbohydrates: 2g / Fiber: 0g

Ingredients:

- 4 salmon fillets
- 2 tablespoons olive oil
- Zest of one lemon
- 2 tablespoons fresh lemon juice
- 2 tablespoons Dijon mustard
- 1 teaspoon dried dill
- Salt and pepper to taste

Instructions:

1. Preheat the grill to medium-high heat.
2. In a bowl, mix olive oil, lemon zest, lemon juice, Dijon mustard, dried dill, salt, and pepper.
3. Brush the salmon fillets with the lemon Dijon mixture.
4. Grill for 4-5 minutes per side until salmon flakes easily with a fork.
5. Serve immediately.

Nutritional Information:

- Calories: 300
- Protein: 28g
- Fat: 20g
- Carbohydrates: 2g
- Fiber: 0g

3. Spicy Cajun Blackened Catfish

Ingredients:

- 4 catfish fillets
- 2 tablespoons olive oil
- 1 tablespoon Cajun seasoning
- 1 teaspoon paprika
- 1/2 teaspoon garlic powder
- 1/2 teaspoon onion powder
- Salt and pepper to taste

Instructions:

1. Preheat a cast-iron skillet over medium-high heat.
2. In a bowl, mix olive oil, Cajun seasoning, paprika, garlic powder, onion powder, salt, and pepper.
3. Brush the catfish fillets with the spice mixture.
4. Cook for 3-4 minutes per side until blackened and cooked through.
5. Serve with a squeeze of fresh lemon.

Nutritional Information:

- Calories: 250
- Protein: 26g
- Fat: 14g
- Carbohydrates: 1g
- Fiber: 0g

4. Garlic Parmesan Baked Cod

Ingredients:

- 4 cod fillets
- 3 tablespoons unsalted butter, melted
- 3 cloves garlic, minced
- 1/4 cup grated Parmesan cheese
- 1 tablespoon fresh parsley, chopped
- Salt and pepper to taste

Instructions:

1. Preheat the oven to 400°F (200°C).
2. Place cod fillets on a baking sheet.
3. In a bowl, mix melted butter, minced garlic, grated Parmesan, salt, and pepper.
4. Brush the cod fillets with the garlic Parmesan mixture.
5. Bake for 12-15 minutes until fish is opaque and flakes easily.
6. Sprinkle with fresh parsley before serving.

Nutritional Information:

- Calories: 230
- Protein: 28g
- Fat: 12g
- Carbohydrates: 1g
- Fiber: 0g

Ingredients:

- 2 cans tuna in water, drained
- 2 avocados, diced
- 1/4 cup red onion, finely chopped
- 1/4 cup celery, diced
- 2 tablespoons mayonnaise
- 1 tablespoon Dijon mustard
- Salt and pepper to taste

Instructions:

1. In a bowl, mix drained tuna, diced avocados, chopped red onion, and diced celery.
2. In a small bowl, whisk together mayonnaise, Dijon mustard, salt, and pepper.
3. Add the dressing to the tuna mixture and toss gently.
4. Serve chilled on a bed of lettuce or as a sandwich.

Nutritional Information:

- Calories: 320
- Protein: 28g
- Fat: 20g
- Carbohydrates: 8g
- Fiber: 6g

Adjust portion sizes based on individual dietary needs and preferences.

WEEKLY MEAL PLANS FOR EASY ADHERENCE.

Here's a 28-days weekly meal plan for the Atkins Diet. Keep in mind that individual dietary needs may vary, so feel free to adjust portion sizes and food choices based on your preferences and nutritional requirements.

Let's create a diverse and delicious weekly meal plan using the recipes provided:

Monday:

Breakfast:

- Scrambled eggs with spinach and feta cheese cooked in butter
- Bulletproof coffee with heavy cream

Lunch:

- Grilled chicken Caesar salad with bacon and Parmesan cheese
- Sugar-free iced tea

Dinner:

- Baked salmon with lemon and dill
- Steamed broccoli with garlic butter

Tuesday:

Breakfast:

- Greek yogurt with berries and a sprinkle of chia seeds

Lunch:

- Cobb salad with turkey, avocado, blue cheese, and ranch dressing

Dinner:

- Zucchini noodles with pesto and grilled shrimp
- Mixed green salad with olive oil dressing

Wednesday:

Breakfast:

- Keto smoothie with almond milk, spinach, avocado, and protein powder

Lunch:

- Egg salad lettuce wraps with mayonnaise and mustard
- Sliced cucumber on the side

Dinner:

- Beef stir-fry with broccoli, bell peppers, and soy sauce
- Cauliflower rice

Thursday:

Breakfast:

- Omelette with mushrooms, cheese, and herbs
- Black coffee

Lunch:

- Tuna salad stuffed bell peppers with cream cheese
- Sugar-free iced tea

Dinner:

- Grilled pork chops with rosemary and garlic
- Roasted Brussels sprouts with bacon

Friday:

Breakfast:

- Keto pancakes with sugar-free syrup and a side of berries

Lunch:

- Caprese salad with cherry tomatoes, mozzarella, and basil
- Avocado slices drizzled with balsamic glaze

Dinner:

- Shrimp and broccoli Alfredo with shirataki noodles

Saturday:

Breakfast:

- Smoked salmon and cream cheese roll-ups
- Bulletproof coffee with MCT oil

Lunch:

- Chicken avocado lettuce wraps with salsa
- Sliced radishes on the side

Dinner:

- Grilled steak with garlic butter
- Asparagus spears roasted in olive oil

Sunday:

Breakfast:

- Chia seed pudding made with almond milk and topped with nuts and seeds

Lunch:

- Turkey and cheese roll-ups with mayo and mustard
- Celery sticks with cream cheese

Dinner:

- Baked chicken thighs with lemon and herbs
- Sauteed spinach with garlic

Week 2:

Monday:

Breakfast:

- Scrambled eggs with spinach and feta cheese cooked in butter
- Bulletproof coffee with heavy cream

Lunch:

- Grilled chicken Caesar salad with bacon and Parmesan cheese
- Sugar-free iced tea

Dinner:

- Zucchini noodles with pesto and grilled shrimp
- Mixed green salad with olive oil dressing

Tuesday:

Breakfast:

- Greek yogurt with berries and a sprinkle of chia seeds

Lunch:

- Egg salad lettuce wraps with mayonnaise and mustard
- Sliced cucumber on the side

Dinner:

- Beef stir-fry with broccoli, bell peppers, and soy sauce
- Cauliflower rice

Wednesday:

Breakfast:

- Omelette with mushrooms, cheese, and herbs
- Black coffee

Lunch:

- Tuna salad stuffed bell peppers with cream cheese
- Sugar-free iced tea

Dinner:

- Shrimp and broccoli Alfredo with shirataki noodles

Thursday:

Breakfast:

- Keto pancakes with sugar-free syrup and a side of berries

Lunch:

- Caprese salad with cherry tomatoes, mozzarella, and basil
- Avocado slices drizzled with balsamic glaze

Dinner:

- Grilled pork chops with rosemary and garlic
- Roasted Brussels sprouts with bacon

Friday:

Breakfast:

- Smoked salmon and cream cheese roll-ups
- Bulletproof coffee with MCT oil

Lunch:

- Chicken avocado lettuce wraps with salsa
- Sliced radishes on the side

Dinner:

- Lemon Garlic Butter Shrimp Scampi
- Zucchini noodles on the side

Saturday:

Breakfast:

- Keto smoothie with almond milk, spinach, avocado, and protein powder

Lunch:

- Cobb salad with turkey, avocado, blue cheese, and ranch dressing

Dinner:

- Grilled steak with garlic butter
- Asparagus spears roasted in olive oil

Sunday:

Breakfast:

- Chia seed pudding made with almond milk and topped with nuts and seeds

Lunch:

- Turkey and cheese roll-ups with mayo and mustard
- Celery sticks with cream cheese

Dinner:

- Garlic Parmesan Baked Cod
- Steamed broccoli with butter

Monday:

Breakfast:

- Keto pancakes with sugar-free syrup and a side of berries

Lunch:

- Grilled chicken Caesar salad with bacon and Parmesan cheese
- Sugar-free iced tea

Dinner:

- Beef stir-fry with broccoli, bell peppers, and soy sauce
- Cauliflower rice

Tuesday:

Breakfast:

- Omelette with mushrooms, cheese, and herbs
- Black coffee

Lunch:

- Tuna salad stuffed bell peppers with cream cheese
- Sugar-free iced tea

Dinner:

- Lemon Garlic Butter Shrimp Scampi
- Zucchini noodles on the side

Wednesday:

Breakfast:

- Greek yogurt with berries and a sprinkle of chia seeds

Lunch:

- Caprese salad with cherry tomatoes, mozzarella, and basil
- Avocado slices drizzled with balsamic glaze

Dinner:

- Grilled pork chops with rosemary and garlic
- Roasted Brussels sprouts with bacon

Thursday:

Breakfast:

- Smoked salmon and cream cheese roll-ups
- Bulletproof coffee with MCT oil

Lunch:

- Chicken avocado lettuce wraps with salsa
- Sliced radishes on the side

Dinner:

- Zucchini Noodles with Pesto and Cherry Tomatoes
- Mixed green salad with olive oil dressing

Friday:

Breakfast:

- Chia seed pudding made with almond milk and topped with nuts and seeds

Lunch:

- Cobb salad with turkey, avocado, blue cheese, and ranch dressing

Dinner:

- Garlic Parmesan Baked Cod
- Steamed broccoli with butter

Saturday:

Breakfast:

- Keto smoothie with almond milk, spinach, avocado, and protein powder

Lunch:

- Egg salad lettuce wraps with mayonnaise and mustard
- Sliced cucumber on the side

Dinner:

- Shrimp and Broccoli Alfredo with Shirataki Noodles

Sunday:

Breakfast:

- Scrambled eggs with spinach and feta cheese cooked in butter
- Bulletproof coffee with heavy cream

Lunch:

- Turkey and cheese roll-ups with mayo and mustard
- Celery sticks with cream cheese

Dinner:

- Grilled Lemon Dijon Salmon
- Asparagus spears roasted in olive oil

Week 4:

Monday:

Breakfast:

- Scrambled eggs with spinach and feta cheese cooked in butter
- Bulletproof coffee with heavy cream

Lunch:

- Chicken avocado lettuce wraps with salsa
- Sliced radishes on the side

Dinner:

- Grilled Lemon Garlic Shrimp Skewers
- Zucchini noodles with pesto

Tuesday:

Breakfast:

- Greek yogurt with berries and a sprinkle of chia seeds

Lunch:

- Caprese salad with cherry tomatoes, mozzarella, and basil
- Avocado slices drizzled with balsamic glaze

Dinner:

- Beef stir-fry with broccoli, bell peppers, and soy sauce
- Cauliflower rice

Wednesday:

Breakfast:

- Keto pancakes with sugar-free syrup and a side of berries

Lunch:

- Tuna salad stuffed bell peppers with cream cheese
- Sugar-free iced tea

Dinner:

- Garlic Parmesan Baked Cod
- Steamed broccoli with butter

Thursday:

Breakfast:

- Omelette with mushrooms, cheese, and herbs
- Black coffee

Lunch:

- Grilled chicken Caesar salad with bacon and Parmesan cheese
- Sugar-free iced tea

Dinner:

- Shrimp and Broccoli Alfredo with Shirataki Noodles

Friday:

Breakfast:

- Smoked salmon and cream cheese roll-ups
- Bulletproof coffee with MCT oil

Lunch:

- Cobb salad with turkey, avocado, blue cheese, and ranch dressing

Dinner:

- Zucchini Noodles with Pesto and Cherry Tomatoes
- Mixed green salad with olive oil dressing

Saturday:

Breakfast:

- Keto smoothie with almond milk, spinach, avocado, and protein powder

Lunch:

- Egg salad lettuce wraps with mayonnaise and mustard
- Sliced cucumber on the side

Dinner:

- Grilled pork chops with rosemary and garlic
- Roasted Brussels sprouts with bacon

Sunday:

Breakfast:

- Chia seed pudding made with almond milk and topped with nuts and seeds

Lunch:

- Turkey and cheese roll-ups with mayo and mustard
- Celery sticks with cream cheese

Dinner:

- Grilled Lemon Dijon Salmon
- Asparagus spears roasted in olive oil

Remember to stay hydrated throughout the day and listen to your body's hunger and fullness cues. If you have any specific dietary restrictions or health concerns, it's always a good idea to consult with a healthcare professional or a registered dietitian before starting any new diet plan.

CHAPTER FIVE
PROTEIN AND FATS ESSENTIALS

Understanding the Role of Protein and Healthy Fats in the Diet

In the intricate dance of nutrition, protein and healthy fats take center stage, playing vital roles in sustaining our health and well-being. Understanding the unique contributions of these macronutrients empowers us to make informed dietary choices, shaping a foundation for vitality and longevity.

Protein's Crucial Role:

Protein, often referred to as the body's building block, serves a plethora of functions essential for life. Comprising amino acids, the body utilizes protein to build and repair tissues, create enzymes and hormones, and support immune function. From the cellular level to the outward structure of muscles, skin, and hair, protein is omnipresent and indispensable.

In the context of weight management, protein takes on a particularly strategic role. Its high thermic effect means that the body expends more energy digesting and metabolizing protein compared to fats and carbohydrates. This, in turn, can contribute to a feeling of fullness, potentially aiding in weight loss and weight maintenance. For those engaging in physical activities, protein becomes a key player in muscle repair and growth, supporting athletic endeavors and promoting overall fitness.

Navigating Healthy Fats:

Contrary to the once-prevailing notion that fats are the enemy, modern nutritional science champions the importance of healthy fats in a balanced diet. Fats, like protein, are crucial for various bodily functions. They serve as a concentrated source of energy, insulate organs, and facilitate the absorption of fat-soluble vitamins (A, D, E, and K). Beyond these fundamental roles, the type of fats we consume matters significantly.

Distinguishing between healthy and unhealthy fats is imperative for optimal well-being. Monounsaturated fats, found in olive oil, avocados, and nuts, have been associated with heart health and may help regulate cholesterol levels. Polyunsaturated fats, including omega-3 and omega-6 fatty acids, play a role in brain function, reduce inflammation, and support cardiovascular health. Sources of these beneficial fats include fatty fish, flaxseeds, and walnuts.

Conversely, saturated fats, prevalent in animal products and some tropical oils, and trans fats, often found in processed and fried foods, are associated with an increased risk of heart disease. Recognizing the distinction between healthy and unhealthy fats empowers individuals to make dietary choices aligned with long-term health goals.

Practical Tips for Balanced Nutrition

Amidst the abundance of dietary advice and ever-evolving trends, achieving balanced nutrition might seem like a daunting task. However, with practical tips and a mindful approach, crafting a well-rounded, nutrient-dense diet becomes not only feasible but also enjoyable.

Prioritize Whole Foods:

At the core of balanced nutrition lies a focus on whole, minimally processed foods. These include a variety of fruits, vegetables, lean proteins, whole grains, and healthy fats. Whole foods provide a spectrum of essential nutrients, including vitamins, minerals, fiber, and antioxidants, promoting overall health and reducing the risk of chronic diseases.

By incorporating a rainbow of fruits and vegetables into your meals, you ensure a diverse array of nutrients, each with its unique health benefits. Choose whole grains over refined grains for added fiber and sustained energy. Opt for lean protein sources such as poultry, fish, beans, and legumes to meet your body's protein needs without excessive saturated fat.

Mindful Portion Control:

While the quality of your food choices matters, so does the quantity. Portion control is a fundamental aspect of balanced nutrition, preventing overconsumption of calories and fostering a healthy relationship with food. Adopting mindful eating practices, such as paying attention to hunger and fullness cues, can help you maintain a harmonious balance.

Consider using smaller plates to create visual cues for appropriate portion sizes. Chew your food slowly, savoring each bite, and allowing your body time to signal satiety. Listen to your body's cues of hunger and fullness, distinguishing between physical hunger and emotional eating. Cultivating a mindful approach to meals promotes a positive relationship with food and encourages sustainable, healthful eating habits.

Strategic Meal Planning:

In the hustle and bustle of daily life, the convenience of fast food and pre-packaged meals can be tempting. However, investing time in strategic meal planning pays dividends in terms of health and nutrition. By planning your meals ahead of time, you gain control over ingredients, portions, and nutritional content.

Start by outlining a weekly meal plan that includes a variety of foods from different food groups. Prepare shopping lists based on your meal plan to avoid impulse purchases and ensure your kitchen is stocked with wholesome ingredients. Batch cooking on weekends can save time during busy weekdays, providing you with nutritious, home-cooked options even on hectic days.

Balancing Macronutrients:

A well-balanced diet involves not only the quality and quantity of food but also the distribution of macronutrients—protein, fats, and carbohydrates. While individual needs vary, a general guideline for balanced macronutrient intake is to derive about 20-35% of your daily calories from fats, 10-35% from protein, and 45-65% from carbohydrates.

Include a source of protein in each meal to support muscle health and satiety. Choose healthy fats, such as avocados, nuts, and olive oil, to fulfill your body's energy needs. Incorporate complex carbohydrates like whole grains, fruits, and vegetables for sustained energy and a rich source of vitamins and minerals.

Hydration Matters:

Often overlooked but undeniably crucial, adequate hydration is a cornerstone of balanced nutrition. Water plays a vital role in digestion, nutrient absorption, temperature regulation, and overall cellular function. Dehydration can lead to fatigue, impaired cognitive function, and even an increased perception of hunger.

Ensure you're consuming an adequate amount of water throughout the day. While individual hydration needs vary, a general recommendation is around eight 8-ounce glasses of water per day. Adjust your intake based on factors such as physical activity, climate, and individual preferences. Infuse water with slices of fruits or herbs to add flavor without the added sugars found in many commercial beverages.

Moderation, Not Deprivation:

Balanced nutrition is not synonymous with deprivation. It's about making choices that nourish your body while allowing room for enjoyment. Indulging in occasional treats or favorite foods is a natural part of a healthy relationship with food. The key lies in moderation and mindful consumption.

Acknowledge that no food is inherently good or bad. Rather than labeling foods, view your diet holistically, considering the overall pattern of your eating habits. Embrace the 80/20 rule, focusing on nutrient-dense, whole foods 80% of the time while leaving room for flexibility and enjoyment in the remaining 20%. This approach fosters a sustainable and realistic approach to balanced nutrition.

In conclusion, the essence of balanced nutrition lies in a holistic and mindful approach to eating. By understanding the roles of protein and healthy fats, prioritizing whole foods, practicing portion control, strategic meal planning, balancing macronutrients, staying hydrated, and embracing moderation, individuals can cultivate a sustainable and health-promoting relationship with food. These practical tips serve as a compass, guiding you on a journey toward optimal well-being through the power of balanced nutrition.

CHAPTER SIX
OVERCOMING COMMON HURDLES

Addressing Plateaus and Dealing with Cravings

Embarking on a journey toward a healthier lifestyle often comes with its share of challenges, and two common hurdles that many individuals encounter are plateaus in progress and the persistent presence of cravings. While these obstacles may seem daunting, understanding their roots and implementing effective strategies can pave the way for continued success on your wellness journey.

Understanding Plateaus:

Reaching a plateau in your health and fitness journey is a common occurrence and, surprisingly, can be a sign of progress. When the body adapts to a consistent routine, whether it be in terms of diet or exercise, it becomes more efficient, potentially leading to a temporary standstill in results. Recognizing a plateau as a natural part of the process allows for a more constructive response.

To overcome plateaus, consider introducing variety into your routine. If your workout has become monotonous, try incorporating new exercises or changing the intensity and duration of your sessions. In terms of diet, recalibrate your approach by adjusting macronutrient ratios or experimenting with different nutrient timings. This strategic variation prevents the body from settling into a comfort zone, reigniting progress.

Additionally, reassessing your goals and celebrating non-scale victories, such as improved energy levels or enhanced mood, can shift the focus from a numeric target to the holistic benefits of a healthy lifestyle. Plateaus are not roadblocks but rather opportunities for adaptation and growth.

Strategies for Tackling Cravings:

Cravings, often intense desires for specific foods, can pose a considerable challenge to maintaining a balanced and healthy diet. While succumbing to cravings occasionally is a normal part of life, persistent or overwhelming cravings may require strategic interventions to prevent them from derailing your progress.

Understanding the root cause of cravings is the first step in managing them effectively. Cravings can be triggered by various factors, including emotional states, hormonal fluctuations, or dietary imbalances. By identifying the specific cues that lead to cravings, you can tailor your approach to address them at the source.

One effective strategy is to ensure your meals are well-balanced and satisfying. Including a mix of macronutrients—protein, fats, and carbohydrates—provides sustained energy and helps prevent the rapid spikes and crashes in blood sugar that can contribute to cravings. Additionally, staying hydrated is crucial, as thirst can often be mistaken for hunger.

Mindful eating practices, such as paying attention to hunger and fullness cues, can also be instrumental in managing cravings. Slow down during meals, savor each bite, and listen to your body's signals. This approach fosters a more conscious and intentional relationship with food, reducing the likelihood of impulsive or emotional eating.

In instances where cravings persist, consider incorporating healthier alternatives. If you're craving something sweet, opt for fresh fruits or a small serving of dark chocolate. Craving salty snacks? Choose a handful of nuts or seeds. Finding nutritious substitutes allows you to satisfy your cravings while still aligning with your health goals.

Lastly, addressing the emotional component of cravings is crucial. Stress, boredom, and other emotions can trigger cravings as a coping mechanism. Developing alternative strategies for managing stress, such as exercise, meditation, or engaging in a favorite hobby, can redirect the focus away from food as a comfort mechanism.

Strategies for Social Situations and Dining Out

Navigating social situations and dining out while adhering to a specific dietary plan can present unique challenges. The abundance of tempting choices, peer influence, and the desire to indulge can make these situations potential stumbling blocks. However, with strategic planning and a mindful approach, you can enjoy social interactions without compromising your health and wellness goals.

Strategic Preparations for Social Situations:

Social gatherings often revolve around food, and preparing for these occasions is key to staying on track. One effective strategy is to eat a balanced and satisfying meal before attending an event. Arriving satiated reduces the likelihood of succumbing to unhealthy snacks or overindulging in less nutritious options.

Communicating your dietary preferences or restrictions with friends and family can also be beneficial. Many hosts appreciate knowing in advance about any dietary considerations, allowing them to accommodate your needs. This proactive communication ensures you have options aligned with your health goals, fostering a more enjoyable experience for everyone involved.

If appropriate, consider bringing a dish to share that aligns with your dietary preferences. Not only does this guarantee a wholesome option for you, but it also introduces others to delicious and nutritious alternatives. Potluck-style gatherings offer a variety of choices, making it easier for everyone to find something they enjoy.

Mindful Choices When Dining Out:

Dining out poses its own set of challenges, but with a strategic and mindful approach, you can savor the experience while making choices that align with your health goals.

Start by reviewing the menu in advance, when possible. Many restaurants now provide their menus online, allowing you to assess the available options and make informed choices. Look for dishes that incorporate lean proteins, vegetables, and whole grains.

When ordering, don't hesitate to customize your meal. Requesting substitutions or modifications to meet your dietary preferences is a common practice and is generally well-received by restaurant staff. For example, opting for a side salad or extra vegetables instead of fries can enhance the nutritional profile of your meal.

Portion control is crucial when dining out, as restaurant servings are often larger than necessary. Consider sharing dishes with a friend or opting for an appetizer and a side instead of a full entrée. If portions are generous, practice mindful eating by stopping when you feel satisfied and requesting a to-go container for leftovers.

Alcohol can contribute additional calories and may lower inhibitions, potentially leading to less mindful eating. If you choose to consume alcohol, do so in moderation, and consider interspersing alcoholic beverages with water to stay hydrated.

In social situations where food is abundant, prioritize engaging in conversations and activities. Redirecting your focus from the buffet or appetizer table can help mitigate the temptation to continuously graze.

Additionally, savor each bite and eat slowly, allowing your body time to signal fullness.

Handling Peer Influence:

Social situations often involve peer influence, and managing external pressures is crucial to staying true to your health goals. One effective strategy is to communicate assertively about your dietary choices without being confrontational. Expressing your commitment to a healthy lifestyle and the positive impact it has on your well-being can garner support and understanding.

If you encounter resistance or skepticism, remember that your health is a personal choice. Focus on the positive changes you've experienced and emphasize that your choices are aligned with your individual goals. Educating others about your dietary preferences can dispel misconceptions and foster a supportive environment.

In conclusion, overcoming common hurdles such as plateaus and cravings requires a combination of understanding the underlying factors and implementing effective strategies. By recognizing plateaus as opportunities for adaptation and addressing cravings through mindful eating and balanced nutrition, individuals can navigate these challenges successfully. Similarly, strategic preparations for social situations and mindful choices when dining out empower individuals to enjoy these occasions while staying aligned with their health and wellness goals. With a proactive and intentional approach, these common hurdles become stepping stones toward sustained well-being and a fulfilling lifestyle.

Exploring Benefits for Cardiovascular Health, Blood Sugar Control, and More

The Atkins Diet, renowned for its low-carbohydrate approach, extends beyond its association with weight loss. Delving into the intricacies of this dietary regimen unveils a myriad of potential benefits that extend to cardiovascular health, blood sugar control, and various aspects of overall well-being.

Cardiovascular Health:

One of the notable and often studied benefits of the Atkins Diet is its potential positive impact on cardiovascular health. Contrary to early concerns about the effects of high-fat diets on heart health, emerging research suggests that the Atkins Diet may contribute to favorable changes in cardiovascular risk factors.

The diet's emphasis on healthy fats, such as monounsaturated and polyunsaturated fats, found in olive oil, avocados, and fatty fish, aligns with current understanding regarding heart-healthy dietary patterns. These fats have been associated with improvements in cholesterol levels, particularly by increasing high-density lipoprotein (HDL or "good" cholesterol) while reducing levels of low-density lipoprotein (LDL or "bad" cholesterol).

Additionally, the Atkins Diet's potential to aid in weight loss can indirectly benefit cardiovascular health. Excess weight, particularly visceral fat, is a known risk factor for heart disease. By promoting weight loss and reducing inflammation associated with obesity, the Atkins Diet may contribute to an overall reduction in cardiovascular risk.

Blood Sugar Control:

For individuals grappling with issues related to blood sugar control, the Atkins Diet presents a promising avenue for management. The low-carbohydrate nature of the diet is particularly advantageous for those with insulin resistance, prediabetes, or type 2 diabetes.

By limiting the intake of carbohydrates, the Atkins Diet minimizes the post-meal spikes in blood sugar levels that can challenge insulin sensitivity. This controlled approach to carbohydrate consumption can lead to more stable blood sugar levels, reducing the need for large insulin releases and potentially aiding in glycemic control.

Research indicates that the Atkins Diet may be effective in improving insulin sensitivity and glycemic control in individuals with type 2 diabetes. However, those with diabetes or other metabolic conditions must work closely with healthcare professionals when considering dietary changes, ensuring that adjustments align with individual health needs.

Weight Loss and Beyond:

While weight loss is often the initial motivator for individuals embarking on the Atkins Diet, the benefits extend beyond shedding excess pounds. The reduction in carbohydrate intake induces a state of ketosis, where the body shifts from utilizing glucose as its primary fuel source to burning fat for energy.

This metabolic shift not only aids in weight loss but also has potential cognitive benefits. Some studies suggest that ketones, produced during ketosis, may have neuroprotective properties and could offer therapeutic advantages for conditions such as epilepsy and neurodegenerative disorders.

Beyond the physical aspects, many individuals report improvements in energy levels, mental clarity, and mood when following the Atkins Diet. Stable blood sugar levels and the avoidance of energy crashes associated with high-carbohydrate diets contribute to sustained energy throughout the day.

Tips for Transitioning Between Phases and Maintaining Results

As individuals progress through the different phases of the Atkins Diet, from Induction to Maintenance, a thoughtful and strategic approach becomes paramount. Successfully transitioning between phases and maintaining the results achieved requires attention to dietary adjustments, lifestyle choices, and ongoing self-awareness.

Smooth Transition Between Phases:

Transitioning from one phase of the Atkins Diet to another involves a gradual adjustment of macronutrient intake, allowing the body to adapt and avoid potential side effects. Here are some tips for navigating these transitions seamlessly:

1. **Gradual Carbohydrate Increase:** During the transition from the Induction Phase to subsequent phases, gradually increase your daily carbohydrate intake. This measured approach helps prevent rapid weight regain and allows your body to adjust to higher levels of carbohydrates without disrupting the state of ketosis abruptly.

2. **Monitor Your Body's Response:** Pay close attention to how your body responds to changes in carbohydrate intake. Track your energy levels, mood, and any changes in weight or body composition. This self-monitoring helps you make informed decisions about the ideal carbohydrate balance for your individual needs.

3. **Incorporate a Variety of Foods:** Embrace the opportunity to incorporate a wider variety of foods

as you progress through the phases. Explore new vegetables, fruits, and whole grains to ensure a diverse and nutrient-rich diet. This diversity not only contributes to overall health but also enhances the sustainability of the Atkins lifestyle.

4. **Reassess Macronutrient Ratios:** As you move through the phases, reassess your macronutrient ratios to find a balance that supports your health goals. While the early phases emphasize higher fat and moderate protein intake, the Maintenance Phase encourages a more balanced distribution of macronutrients to support long-term sustainability.

Maintaining Results:

Sustaining the results achieved on the Atkins Diet involves more than just adhering to dietary guidelines. Lifestyle factors, ongoing self-awareness, and a holistic approach to health play crucial roles in maintaining long-term success:

1. **Lifestyle Choices Matter:** Beyond dietary considerations, lifestyle choices significantly impact the maintenance of results. Regular physical activity, adequate sleep, stress management, and hydration contribute to overall well-being and support the metabolic advantages of the Atkins Diet.

2. **Regular Exercise Routine:** Engage in a regular exercise routine that aligns with your fitness goals. Physical activity not only aids in weight management but also promotes cardiovascular health, muscle tone, and overall vitality. Choose activities you enjoy to enhance adherence and sustainability.

3. **Mindful Eating Practices:** Cultivate mindful eating practices to maintain a conscious and intentional

approach to meals. Pay attention to hunger and fullness cues, savor each bite, and be present during meals. Mindful eating fosters a positive relationship with food and reduces the likelihood of overeating.

4. **Regular Health Check-ups:** Schedule regular health check-ups with healthcare professionals to monitor key health indicators, including cholesterol levels, blood pressure, and blood sugar. These assessments provide valuable insights into your overall health and allow for timely adjustments if needed.

5. **Adapt to Changing Needs:** Recognize that your nutritional and lifestyle needs may evolve. Life circumstances, age, and health considerations can influence your dietary requirements. Stay attuned to your body's signals and be open to adjusting your approach to align with changing needs.

6. **Cultivate a Supportive Environment:** Surround yourself with a supportive environment that aligns with your health goals. Share your journey with friends, family, or a community of like-minded individuals. Having a supportive network can provide encouragement, accountability, and a sense of camaraderie.

7. **Celebrate Non-scale Victories:** Beyond the numbers on the scale, celebrate non-scale victories that reflect improvements in overall well-being. Whether it's increased energy levels, enhanced mood, or achieving fitness milestones, acknowledging these achievements reinforces the positive impact of your lifestyle choices.

In conclusion, the Atkins Diet offers a multifaceted approach to health, encompassing benefits for cardiovascular health, blood sugar control, weight management, and overall well-being. Navigating the transitions between phases and maintaining results involves a combination of strategic dietary adjustments, lifestyle choices, and ongoing self-awareness. By embracing the holistic principles of the Atkins lifestyle, individuals can experience sustained health benefits and cultivate a fulfilling and enduring approach to wellness.

CHAPTER EIGHT
INTEGRATING EXERCISE

Importance of Physical Activity in Conjunction with the Atkins Diet

The synergy between the Atkins Diet and regular physical activity forms a powerful alliance in the pursuit of overall health and well-being. While the Atkins Diet lays the foundation for effective weight management and metabolic health, integrating exercise into the equation amplifies these benefits and contributes to a holistic approach to fitness.

Weight Management and Beyond:

Physical activity serves as a dynamic companion to the Atkins Diet, especially when it comes to weight management. While the low-carbohydrate approach of the diet addresses the metabolic aspect of weight loss, exercise enhances the caloric expenditure side of the equation. The combination of dietary modifications and increased physical activity creates a more comprehensive strategy for achieving and maintaining a healthy weight.

Engaging in regular exercise not only burns calories but also contributes to the preservation of lean muscle mass—a key component of a healthy metabolism. As individuals follow the Atkins Diet to reduce carbohydrate intake and enter states of ketosis, incorporating exercise becomes instrumental in optimizing fat utilization for energy.

Enhancing Metabolic Health:

Beyond its impact on weight, physical activity plays a pivotal role in enhancing metabolic health. The Atkins Diet, particularly in its earlier phases, induces a state of ketosis where the body efficiently utilizes fats for energy. Exercise complements this metabolic state by promoting insulin sensitivity and improving glucose utilization.

Research suggests that combining a low-carbohydrate diet with regular exercise may offer synergistic benefits for blood sugar control. Exercise increases the uptake of glucose by muscles, reducing the reliance on insulin for glucose regulation. This collaborative approach can be particularly advantageous for individuals with insulin resistance, prediabetes, or type 2 diabetes.

Cardiovascular Fitness:

Cardiovascular health is a cornerstone of overall well-being, and the integration of exercise further fortifies the benefits of the Atkins Diet. Aerobic exercise, such as walking, jogging, cycling, or swimming, elevates heart rate and respiratory activity, promoting cardiovascular fitness. This not only supports heart health but also enhances endurance and stamina.

While the Atkins Diet has been associated with improvements in cholesterol levels, adding cardiovascular exercise amplifies these benefits. Regular aerobic activity has been shown to raise levels of high-density lipoprotein (HDL or "good" cholesterol) while lowering levels of low-density lipoprotein (LDL or "bad" cholesterol), contributing to a favorable lipid profile.

Mood and Mental Well-being:

Exercise is not solely about physical outcomes—it exerts a profound impact on mental well-being. The release of endorphins, often referred to as "feel-good" hormones, during exercise contributes to improved mood and reduced feelings of stress and anxiety. The mental clarity and cognitive benefits reported by individuals on the Atkins Diet are further enhanced when exercise becomes a consistent part of the routine.

The Atkins Diet's impact on brain function, attributed to the production of ketones during ketosis, aligns harmoniously with the cognitive benefits of regular exercise. Studies suggest that both low-carbohydrate diets and exercise may have neuroprotective effects, potentially reducing the risk of cognitive decline and neurodegenerative disorders.

Tailoring Exercise Routines to Individual Needs

Recognizing that one size does not fit all, tailoring exercise routines to individual needs is a cornerstone of a sustainable and effective fitness strategy. This personalized approach ensures that exercise aligns with individual goals, preferences, and health considerations, fostering long-term adherence and success.

Assessing Individual Goals:

The first step in tailoring an exercise routine is a clear assessment of individual goals. Whether the objective is weight loss, muscle gain, improved cardiovascular health, or a combination of these, defining specific and realistic goals provides a roadmap for designing a targeted exercise plan.

For individuals primarily focused on weight loss in conjunction with the Atkins Diet, a combination of aerobic exercise and resistance training can be beneficial. Aerobic activities burn calories and enhance cardiovascular health, while resistance training contributes to the preservation of lean muscle mass—a critical factor in sustaining a healthy metabolism.

Those aiming for muscle gain or body composition changes may prioritize resistance training, incorporating a mix of exercises targeting different muscle groups. A well-rounded resistance training program, complemented by an adequate protein intake following the principles of the Atkins Diet, supports muscle development and strength.

Considering Health Considerations:

Individual health considerations play a crucial role in shaping an exercise routine that is both safe and effective. Health conditions, previous injuries, and current fitness levels are important factors to consider when tailoring a workout plan.

For individuals with pre-existing health conditions, consultation with healthcare professionals or fitness experts is recommended to ensure that exercise is aligned with medical advice. Modifications and adaptations can be made to accommodate specific health considerations while still providing a beneficial and enjoyable exercise experience.

Previous injuries or areas of vulnerability should be considered when designing an exercise routine. Choosing exercises that minimize impact on sensitive areas, incorporating proper warm-ups and cool-downs, and progressively increasing intensity can help prevent exacerbation of existing issues.

Personal Preferences and Enjoyment:

Sustainable exercise routines are rooted in personal preferences and enjoyment. Tailoring workouts to activities that individuals genuinely enjoy increases the likelihood of adherence and long-term success. Whether it's dancing, hiking, swimming, or weightlifting, finding activities that bring joy and fulfillment transforms exercise from a chore into a rewarding and integral part of daily life.

Varied and engaging workouts also prevent monotony, keeping individuals motivated and excited to stay active. Experimenting with different types of exercise, exploring group classes, or incorporating outdoor activities adds diversity to the routine, making it more enjoyable and sustainable over the long term.

Creating a Realistic Schedule:

Balancing exercise with the demands of daily life requires a realistic and achievable schedule. Tailoring exercise routines to fit individual schedules increases the likelihood of consistency. Whether it's early morning workouts, lunchtime walks, or evening gym sessions, choosing times that align with personal preferences and energy levels fosters adherence.

Shorter, more frequent workouts can be just as effective as longer sessions, especially for individuals with busy schedules. Incorporating physical activity into daily routines, such as taking the stairs, walking during phone calls, or doing quick home workouts, adds up over the course of the day.

Progressive Adaptation:

As fitness levels improve and goals are achieved, a tailored exercise routine should evolve to ensure continued progress. Progressive adaptation involves periodically adjusting the intensity, duration, or type of exercise to challenge the body and prevent plateaus.

Integrating periodization, which involves alternating between periods of higher and lower intensity, can be an effective strategy. This approach prevents burnout, reduces the risk of overtraining, and allows for recovery periods that contribute to overall fitness gains.

In conclusion, integrating exercise with the Atkins Diet enhances the multifaceted benefits of this dietary approach. Recognizing the importance of physical activity for weight management, metabolic health, cardiovascular fitness, and mental well-being underscores the synergistic relationship between diet and exercise. Tailoring exercise routines to individual needs ensures that fitness plans are realistic, enjoyable, and aligned with personal goals and considerations. By embracing a personalized and sustainable approach to exercise, individuals can amplify the positive impact of the Atkins lifestyle on their overall health and vitality.

CHAPTER NINE
YOUR ATKINS TOOLKIT

Supplementary Materials

Embarking on the Atkins Diet journey is akin to setting out on a path toward transformative health. To equip yourself for success, having a well-rounded toolkit of supplementary materials is invaluable. These resources not only enhance your understanding of the Atkins Diet but also provide practical guidance and support throughout your wellness expedition.

Educational Books and Guides:

Foundational knowledge is key to navigating the intricacies of the Atkins Diet. Investing in educational books and guides authored by experts in the field provides comprehensive insights into the principles, phases, and benefits of the diet. These resources often break down complex concepts into digestible information, empowering you with the knowledge needed to make informed choices about your dietary approach.

Look for titles that align with your goals and preferences, whether you're seeking a detailed scientific understanding or a practical guide with recipes and meal plans. Books written by Dr. Robert C. Atkins, the creator of the Atkins Diet, and subsequent editions or publications by reputable nutritionists and dieticians can be valuable additions to your toolkit.

Recipe Books and Cookbooks:

Diversifying your menu while adhering to the principles of the Atkins Diet is made easier with a collection of recipe books and cookbooks. These resources offer creative and delicious low-carb recipes that align with the different phases of the diet. From breakfast options and main courses to snacks and desserts, recipe books inspire crafting satisfying meals without compromising your dietary goals.

Choose books that cater to your taste preferences and dietary restrictions. Whether you're a fan of Mediterranean cuisine, prefer vegetarian options, or are looking for quick and easy recipes for busy days, there are Atkins-friendly cookbooks tailored to various culinary preferences.

Food Journals and Tracking Tools:

Maintaining awareness of your dietary choices is a powerful tool for success. Food journals and tracking tools help you monitor your daily food intake, track your macronutrient ratios, and identify patterns in your eating habits. This self-awareness can be instrumental in adjusting, identifying triggers, and celebrating milestones on your journey.

Opt for physical journals or explore digital tracking apps that streamline the process. Many apps allow you to scan barcodes for easy input of nutritional information and provide visual representations of your dietary patterns over time. Consistent tracking not only supports your adherence to the Atkins Diet but also fosters a deeper understanding of the relationship between your food choices and overall well-being.

Supplemental Reading Materials:

To enrich your understanding of the broader landscape of nutrition, consider including supplemental reading materials in your toolkit. While the Atkins Diet focuses on low-carbohydrate principles, exploring broader topics such as nutritional science, mindful eating, and the role of macronutrients in the body can provide a well-rounded perspective on health and wellness.

Magazines, articles, and online resources from reputable health and nutrition publications can offer ongoing insights and updates. Stay informed about the latest research, trends, and perspectives in the field of nutrition to complement your knowledge base and make informed decisions about your dietary choices.

Shopping Lists

Efficiency in the kitchen begins with strategic planning, and having well-curated shopping lists is the linchpin of a successful Atkins Diet journey. These lists not only streamline your grocery shopping experience but also ensure that your kitchen is stocked with the essential ingredients to create delicious and satisfying low-carb meals.

Foundational Low-Carb Staples:

Crafting a shopping list that includes foundational low-carb staples forms the bedrock of your Atkins toolkit. Items such as lean proteins (poultry, fish, tofu), non-starchy vegetables (leafy greens, broccoli, cauliflower), healthy fats (olive oil, avocados, nuts), and low-carb condiments provide the building blocks for a diverse range of meals across the Atkins Diet phases.

Consider including eggs, dairy or dairy alternatives, and herbs and spices to enhance flavor without relying on high-carb seasonings. Having a consistent supply of these staples ensures that you can whip up satisfying meals while adhering to the principles of the Atkins Diet.

Seasonal and Fresh Produce:

Incorporating seasonal and fresh produce into your shopping list not only adds variety to your meals but also ensures that you benefit from a spectrum of nutrients. Fruits and vegetables with lower carbohydrate content, such as berries, tomatoes, and bell peppers, can be included in moderation as you progress through the diet phases.

Adapt your shopping list based on the seasons to take advantage of the freshest and most flavorful produce.

Familiarize yourself with the carbohydrate content of different fruits and vegetables to make informed choices that align with your dietary goals.

Protein-Rich Snacks and Convenience Foods:

On-the-go options and convenient snacks are integral components of a practical Atkins toolkit. Consider including protein-rich snacks like jerky, hard-boiled eggs, or cheese for quick and satisfying options that align with the low-carb principles of the diet.

Explore the variety of low-carb convenience foods available, such as almond flour, coconut flour, or low-carb wraps, to add flexibility to your meal planning. These items can be particularly useful for creating alternative versions of your favorite recipes without compromising your dietary goals.

Condiments and Sauces:

Elevate the flavor profile of your meals with a selection of low-carb condiments and sauces. Mustard, mayonnaise, hot sauce, and sugar-free ketchup are excellent options to enhance taste without introducing unnecessary carbohydrates.

Read labels carefully to ensure that condiments are free from added sugars and hidden carbs. Having a well-stocked condiment arsenal adds versatility to your meals, allowing you to experiment with flavors and textures while adhering to the Atkins Diet.

Beverages and Hydration Aids:

Staying hydrated is crucial for overall well-being and supports the metabolic processes associated with the Atkins Diet. Include beverages such as water, herbal teas, and sparkling water in your shopping list to maintain adequate hydration throughout the day.

Consider incorporating electrolyte supplements or low-carb sports drinks, especially during the initial phases of the diet when the body is adapting to lower carbohydrate intake. These additions help replenish electrolytes and mitigate potential side effects associated with the transition to ketosis.

Online Resources

The digital age has ushered in a wealth of online resources that can serve as dynamic companions on your Atkins Diet journey. From community support to recipe inspiration, incorporating these online tools into your toolkit enhances accessibility and connectivity in your pursuit of health and wellness.

Official Atkins Website:

The official Atkins website serves as a central hub for a treasure trove of resources tailored to individuals following the Atkins Diet. Comprehensive guides, meal plans, and recipes specific to each phase of the diet are readily available. The website also features success stories, community forums, and expert articles that provide ongoing support and motivation.

Explore the tools and calculators on the website to customize your approach based on individual factors such as age, weight, and activity level. These interactive features can help you fine-tune your dietary plan and set realistic goals throughout your Atkins journey.

Online Community Forums and Support Groups:

Navigating a dietary change is often more enjoyable and sustainable when shared with a community of like-minded individuals. Online forums and support groups dedicated to the Atkins Diet provide a platform for individuals to share experiences, exchange tips, and seek advice from those on similar journeys.

Engaging with an online community fosters a sense of camaraderie and accountability. Whether you have questions about specific phases, need recipe suggestions, or simply want to celebrate milestones, participating in these forums connects you with a supportive network that understands the nuances of the Atkins lifestyle.

Recipe Websites and Blogs:

Diversifying your culinary repertoire is made easy with the plethora of low-carb recipe websites and blogs available online. Explore platforms that curate Atkins-friendly recipes, meal ideas, and cooking tips. Many of these resources provide nutritional information for each recipe, ensuring that you can track your macronutrient intake accurately.

Look for blogs authored by nutritionists, chefs, or individuals who share their personal experiences with the Atkins Diet. These platforms often feature creative adaptations of classic dishes, making it enjoyable to explore new flavors and culinary techniques while staying true to your dietary goals.

Fitness Apps and Trackers:

Incorporate fitness apps and trackers into your online toolkit to streamline the monitoring of physical activity and overall wellness. Many apps allow you to log workouts, track steps, and monitor progress over time. Syncing these tools with wearable devices provides real-time insights into your daily activity levels and supports your fitness goals.

Explore apps that offer guided workouts, personalized fitness plans, and community features. Having a digital record of your exercise achievements adds a motivational element to your fitness journey, encouraging you to stay active and engaged with your health and well-being.

Educational Videos and Webinars:

Visual learners can benefit from educational videos and webinars that delve into the science, benefits, and practical aspects of the Atkins Diet. Platforms such as YouTube often host channels dedicated to low-carb living, featuring content from nutritionists, chefs, and individuals sharing their success stories.

Subscribe to channels that align with your interests and learning style. From cooking demonstrations and meal prep tutorials to in-depth discussions about the physiological aspects of low-carb living, these videos offer a dynamic and engaging supplement to your understanding of the Atkins lifestyle.

Assembling a comprehensive toolkit for your Atkins journey involves gathering supplementary materials, crafting strategic shopping lists, and leveraging the wealth of online resources available. Educational books, recipe guides, and food journals enhance your understanding and implementation of the Atkins Diet principles. Shopping lists ensure that your kitchen is stocked with the essential ingredients for success, and online resources provide ongoing support, community engagement, and inspiration. By integrating these elements into your toolkit, you equip yourself with the knowledge, tools, and connectivity needed to thrive on the Atkins Diet and embrace a lasting journey toward health and well-being.

CONCLUSION

Recap of Key Takeaways

Embarking on the Atkins journey is a transformative step towards a healthier and more vibrant lifestyle. As we conclude this exploration of the Atkins Diet and its multifaceted principles, let's recap the key takeaways that empower you to make informed decisions, embrace a low-carb lifestyle, and experience the potential benefits for your overall well-being.

Understanding the Phases:

The Atkins Diet unfolds in phases, each designed to guide you through a gradual process of carbohydrate reintroduction while promoting sustainable weight loss and metabolic changes. From the Induction Phase, where the focus is on jumpstarting ketosis, to the Maintenance Phase, where a balanced and individualized approach takes center stage, understanding these phases is pivotal.

In the initial phases, emphasis on high-fat and moderate-protein intake prompts the body to shift from using glucose as its primary fuel source to burning stored fat for energy. As you progress, the gradual reintroduction of carbohydrates allows for personalization, ensuring that the diet aligns with your lifestyle, preferences, and health goals.

Balancing Macronutrients:

The Atkins Diet places a spotlight on the importance of balancing macronutrients—fats, proteins, and carbohydrates. Contrary to conventional dietary wisdom, the inclusion of healthy fats is a cornerstone of the Atkins approach. These fats not only provide a sustained source of energy but also contribute to satiety, reducing cravings and promoting a sense of fullness.

Protein plays a crucial role in maintaining lean muscle mass, supporting metabolic health, and aiding in the feeling of satisfaction after meals. By strategically managing carbohydrate intake, the diet minimizes blood sugar spikes, promoting stable energy levels and improved insulin sensitivity.

Embracing Whole Foods:

At the heart of the Atkins Diet is the emphasis on whole, nutrient-dense foods. Non-starchy vegetables, lean proteins, and healthy fats form the foundation of your meals, providing a spectrum of essential vitamins, minerals, and antioxidants. These whole foods not only nourish your body but also contribute to overall health and well-being.

Diversifying your plate with a colorful array of vegetables ensures a rich supply of fiber, promoting digestive health and sustained energy. Incorporating lean proteins supports muscle maintenance and repair, while healthy fats, such as those found in avocados, nuts, and olive oil, offer a host of benefits for cardiovascular health and satiety.

Personalizing Your Approach:

While the Atkins Diet provides a structured framework, personalization is key to long-term success. Your journey is unique, and the flexibility inherent in the diet allows you to tailor your approach based on individual factors such as activity level, health status, and preferences. The phases serve as a guide, but it's the personalized adjustments that make the Atkins Diet a sustainable and enjoyable lifestyle.

Whether you choose to focus on weight loss, blood sugar control, or overall well-being, the Atkins Diet accommodates diverse goals. The ability to adapt and refine your approach as needed ensures that the diet remains a dynamic and supportive tool throughout your health and wellness journey.

Encouragement and Motivation for Readers to Embark on Their Atkins Journey

As you stand at the threshold of your Atkins journey, it's important to embrace the exciting possibilities that lie ahead. Embarking on a new dietary path can be both invigorating and challenging, but the potential for positive transformations in your health and lifestyle is immeasurable. Here, we offer words of encouragement and motivation to propel you forward on your Atkins journey.

Celebrating Progress, Not Perfection:

The Atkins journey is a process of growth, discovery, and positive change. It's essential to approach it with a mindset of progress, not perfection. Every small step, every conscious food choice, and every moment of self-discovery contribute to your overall success.

Celebrate your victories, whether they are scale-related achievements, increased energy levels, or a newfound appreciation for whole foods. Understand that setbacks may occur, and they are merely detours, not roadblocks. The journey is about continuous improvement and the cultivation of a sustainable and fulfilling lifestyle.

Embracing the Learning Curve:

Navigating the Atkins Diet involves a learning curve, and that's perfectly normal. As you explore new recipes, experiment with different food combinations, and understand how your body responds to dietary changes, you're gaining valuable insights into your own wellness.

Embrace the opportunity to learn more about the intricacies of nutrition, the science behind the diet, and how your body thrives on a low-carb approach. Knowledge is empowerment, and the more you understand about the principles of the Atkins Diet, the more confidently you can navigate the diverse phases and personalize your journey.

Cultivating a Positive Relationship with Food:

The Atkins Diet invites you to cultivate a positive and intentional relationship with food. It's not just about what you eat but how you nourish your body and soul. Approach each meal with mindfulness, savoring the flavors, and appreciating the nourishment it provides.

Shift your perspective from restrictive thinking to a mindset of abundance. The Atkins Diet offers a wide variety of delicious and nutritious foods that can be enjoyed in creative and satisfying ways. Embrace the joy of culinary exploration and the discovery of flavors that resonate with your taste preferences.

Building a Supportive Community:

Embarking on the Atkins journey doesn't mean going it alone. Building a supportive community can be a game-changer. Connect with fellow Atkins enthusiasts through online forums, social media groups, or local meetups. Share your experiences, seek advice, and celebrate milestones together.

Having a support system provides encouragement during challenging moments and amplifies the joy during successes. Whether you're sharing recipe ideas, discussing strategies for overcoming hurdles, or simply cheering each other on, a community can be a source of inspiration and motivation throughout your journey.

Focusing on Non-Scale Victories:

While weight loss may be a primary goal for many, it's crucial to recognize and celebrate non-scale victories. Improved energy levels enhanced mental clarity, better sleep, and increased physical fitness are all valuable achievements that contribute to your overall well-being.

Shift your focus from solely numerical goals to holistic indicators of health and vitality. Acknowledge the positive changes in how you feel, move, and experience daily life. These non-scale victories are often the most meaningful and sustainable markers of success on your Atkins journey.

Embracing a Lifelong Wellness Journey:

The Atkins Diet isn't just a temporary fix; it's a gateway to a lifelong wellness journey. Embrace the principles of the diet as foundational pillars that support your ongoing commitment to health. As you progress through the phases, view each phase as a stepping stone toward sustained well-being rather than a destination.

Your wellness journey is dynamic and ever evolving. As your body and lifestyle change, your approach to nutrition and health will naturally adapt. Embrace the ebb and flow of this journey, staying open to new discoveries and refining your habits to align with your evolving needs.

In conclusion, the Atkins journey is an invitation to embark on a path of self-discovery, empowerment, and lasting well-being. Recapitulating the key takeaways reinforces the principles of the diet, providing a foundation for your personalized approach. Encouragement and motivation serve as guiding lights, empowering you to navigate challenges, celebrate victories, and embrace the transformative potential of the Atkins lifestyle. As you set forth on your journey, remember that it's not just about reaching a destination—it's about savoring the richness of each step and cultivating a life of vitality, balance, and joy.